One of our greatest assets is time; don't spend it complaining about where you want to be. Take action to get there.

Contents

Acknowledgements

First, I give special thanks to all of my dear clients who inspire me to do what I do every day. I have been so blessed to get to know each and every one of you on such a personal level. You all have enriched my life and your victories exemplify true strength and commitment. Your stories are powerful and have helped others become inspired to start a wellness journey, as you have. Thank you for sharing and for trusting me to help you along the way.

I have had a world of great help preparing this book. Thank you, Carole, for being a wonderful confidante, close friend, and informal editor. Thank you, Will, for all of your humor and guidance in the beginning of this process. You are by far the most talented ghost-writer I have ever met. I could not have confidently finished this first version of this book series without you.

I give a profound thank you to my husband Jeff who challenges me to be better every day of my life. He is a man of impeccable integrity and strength. I will never know the physical challenges he faces on a daily basis and have the utmost respect for him and for his constant efforts in improving the lives of others. He helps me renew my mind every day and stay focused on what really matters...helping people. Thank you, Jeff, for believing in me and all the "risks" I take. None of this is possible without you.

A special note of gratitude is due to my gym family. The

people we employ within our health club believe in the fact that machines don't change people--*people* change people. Our team lives by this principle and allows every member of our health club to be touched daily by a warm smile or a simple act of kindness. We accomplish many things knowing that the whole is greater than its parts. A special thank you goes to my daughter, Hailey. She is a remarkable person and beautiful in so many ways. Thank you, for all you do to make each and every day successful and enjoyable.

To my kids, Hailey and Christian. I love you more than words can ever say. Your unconditional love, patience, and understanding over the years has been amazing. You bring me joy and peace.

And finally, to all my faithful family and friends; keep believing in His Strength, Power, and Energy.

Wisdom is choosing to do now what you will be satisfied with later.

Introduction

If you are ready to change your life, feel better, and become more powerful in everything you do, then your journey starts now. It is time we get back to the basics of good nutrition and not complicate the process of becoming healthier. When we dedicate ourselves to learning more about eating well, extraordinary things begin to happen. We all have the inner strength to reach our goals. The challenge is to learn more so we can harness the *power* of our potential and become the *amazing* people we only dream we can be!

The Fitness Industry – Dream-Makers or Dream-Takers?

Throughout my life, my passion has been fitness. Professionally, I have worked in the fitness industry for over 25 years and have witnessed many changes. During this time I have seen diet and training trends come and go, infomercials and videos come in and out of vogue, dreams and goals achieved and destroyed.

In fact, the fitness industry itself, such an integral part of my life, can be held accountable for some of these dreams and goals not being achieved. Why? It has deceived consumers to think "real" fitness and good health comes in the form of rock hard abs, chiseled muscles, and 2% body fat. Just glance at the cover of a popular fitness magazine. By showcasing images of spectacularly-toned male and female bodies, they imply *this* body defines fitness and optimal health. To achieve this "fit" body, just follow a special diet program for a few weeks, maybe one that offers a "fat-dissolving" pill, protein supplement, magic pills, or formulas that promise you will have the body on the cover with no permanent change to your life. To be honest, we all want someone to tell us, "You can be healthy, happy, and fit without any real discipline."

These slick advertisers know how to catch their prey. After watching infomercials or reading about the latest fad diet, you can easily fall victim to their false promises. Sure, they succeed in motivating you, but only long enough to purchase their products and give them a try.

So what happens? After weeks of taking pills, working out hard and sweating like you never had before, you take a look in the mirror and surprise--you still don't look like the super model on the cover of *Health and Fitness* magazine. Now you really become discouraged and give up.

What motivates you?

Months may pass before you may try to lose weight again, but often you are even more disappointed. Why? One reason may lie in what motivated you to lose weight in the first place. If the motivation was just vanity--"I want to lose weight to *look different*"--the inspiration will be short-lived. Eating well to look different will never keep you motivated for long. Eating well to look different may inspire you to eat well for a couple of weeks, but it will never last a lifetime. You will only achieve life-long results when you finally eat well for reasons that are not just geared to changing the physical body, but the whole being.

Choosing to eat differently to achieve overall *wellness* is the key to changing your nutritional habits for a lifetime. Achieving good health and fitness does not have to be complicated. Simply changing your eating patterns will allow you to feel and perform your best. To help you siphon through the misconceptions and help you reach, and finally maintain, a life full of vitality and strength, I have developed a program called *The Amazing Power of Food.* This program combines simple and easy guidelines with common sense advice on how to become and how to remain healthy, so you have the *power* to reach your *amazing* potential.

Why *The Amazing Power of Food?*

Why am I so convinced *The Amazing Power of Food* works? I have seen the results! To begin, I own a fitness center in Hammond, Louisiana. Every day I see the need for a common sense approach to wellness with my business and our community. I have witnessed numerous failed attempts at dieting and have seen people take desperate, pill popping measures to lose weight. I have seen too many people destroy their health by these desperate measures and in turn destroy their lives. I know results can be achieved by simply eating healthier foods and overcome illness, obesity, addictions, and much more. I have hundreds of case studies that prove this program works. I continually strive to make a positive impact on people by teaching them how vital their health is to their families, employers, and bank accounts. The people who have put this information and meal plan into action not only become healthier, they begin to thrive, not just survive. *The Amazing Power of Food* is a tried and true meal plan that is simple and understandable. I have seen *The Amazing Power of Food* work for many people and I know it can work for you, too. The information you will learn in this book will set you on the path toward complete well-being. After reading the simple guidelines provided in the following chapters, you will discover the radiance within yourself that "diet" and fitness programs alone simply can't provide.

So how does *The Amazing Power of Food* work? People LEARN that the core of good health is good nutrition, not a fad diet. They LEARN that reaching their health and fitness goals can be achieved through GOOD NUTRITION.

The Amazing Power of Food—

As a health and fitness consultant for over 20 years, I have met with hundreds of clients, providing whatever training and counseling they request. They come to me daily, complaining because they are either exercising often and not achieving the results they want or frustrated because they are sick and tired of feeling sick and tired. I know that giving clients a menu to follow for a finite amount of time will not work long term. My desire is to help people create life-long changes regarding their health.

For the last ten years I have witnessed *The Amazing Power of Food* program help people regain their lives: they lose weight and maintain their weight loss; improve blood lipid panels and blood pressure readings; eliminate or reduce daily medications;

and most of all, they FEEL GREAT! How? They understand the "why" behind eating the foods their bodies need. They know that healthy recipes are simple and drastic measures are ineffective. They were given simple explanations and followed a simple plan.

Having the time to personally meet with clients one-on-one enables me to examine their eating patterns as well as their schedules. I learn what foods people like, their schedules, what they enjoy eating for lunch, how they like their coffee, what time they go to bed and much more. In our sessions they divulge what they eat every day, which, by the way, is very eye-opening for most people. I find that people never really think about their nutrition, they just eat. This "discovery" process gives me the necessary information I need to be able to help clients succeed in their new journey to wellness.

Unfortunately, books can't meet with you one-on-one. That is why I procrastinated writing a book. I wasn't sure I could transfer the "magic" that happened in each one of these one-on-one sessions to the printed page. But I knew I had to try. I had to discover what specifically made a difference.

Why did all of my clients achieve fantastic results? Perhaps it was their talking about "how" and "what" they ate on a daily basis; maybe it was the simple and easy-to-understand information I provided that just made sense. Maybe they soon realized how fast-food and high sodium levels could kill them. Maybe they just began to eat better almost immediately. Most likely, I think it was a combination of all these things. Regardless of what exactly worked for each person, each client finally won the battle and incorporated healthier eating habits.

After watching one success story unfold after another, I came to the conclusion that I must write this book. It was the only way to reach a wide audience. I knew I could package the words and explanations that had helped so many. My hope is that by reading *The Amazing Power of Food* and following the menus it provides, you will understand the power that food has over your body.

Even though the media and government programs bombard us with information about how to live healthier lives, none of it seems to be helping our population. So many people are unwell; so many people still do not know HOW to take care of themselves. Obesity and diabetes are at record highs. I personally believe people do not succeed because they cannot easily access or understand the volumes of nutritional information available; they do not or cannot connect with the way the material is presented. Hopefully, the information you read in this book will help you understand how easy eating healthy can be and you will attain and retain as much knowledge as possible so you can become a wellness warrior and begin to fight to be fit!

This book is purposefully simple and straightforward. It is designed to be easy to read and easy to understand. There are ten chapters; each chapter complements and builds upon each other. *"Inspiration" shows* us we all need inspiration to fuel our motivation to be healthier. It asks you to find your own personal inspiration. What is it that will keep you motivated on your journey to wellness?

"What Do You Really Want" is the interactive section. Here you will be asked to write down and disclose what you desire for your health. You will also write down and analyze your daily routine. Something happens when you write down or verbalize your actions and recognize what you're really wanting in regards to your physical health. You make discoveries! You come face to face with how you have been living and how you want to live in the future. This section is a rather crucial step on your way to success.

"Keeping Food Choices Simple" de-clutters the numerous books, videos, and programs on fitness and diets that lead people to a state of mass confusion about being healthy and fit. This chapter shows you that eating well can be quite simple and easy to accomplish.

"Identify Your Eating Pattern" helps you recognize what eating category you fall into, so that you can prevent poor eating patterns in the future.

"Eliminate Excuses" is probably my favorite chapter in this book. Excuses prevail in unhealthy people. Here you hear your own voice making excuses for your careless eating habits. Here, however, you learn how to stop making excuses. Life is just too short to live unwell behind the veil of a poor excuse.

"Untie Your Food" will teach you the secret to losing weight and maintaining your weight loss while remaining in good health. You must learn to *live* fully as you lose weight, and live fully as you maintain a healthy weight. If there is one concept in this book that you always practice, I hope it is this one. Learning how to untie your food will allow you to "live" and lose weight or maintain your weight easily for a lifetime. I know this is a big claim, but I have personally witnessed many people master this simple technique and finally remain in constant control of their health.

"You Must Learn More" gives you information you'll need to eat healthier. My favorite saying is, ***"I did what I could with what I knew; when I knew better, I did better."*** This statement is so true. You need to learn more about what you put in your body and why it matters. You will gain a better understanding about the importance of vitamins and minerals; your body does not run properly without essential nutrients. You will learn about micronutrients and uncover why you cannot live a healthy life without them. Consummate dieters will often focus on the little things like fat-free food items or whole-wheat products to try and eat better. Through illustrations and examples, you will learn how to focus on what really matters when you want to become a healthy eater. Here I will also clearly define the dangers of sodium and other small but dangerous food additives.

"Steps to Eating Healthier" gives you meal tips and strategies to eat healthy every day. You will find tips for breakfast, lunch, and dinner, as well as learn the importance of snacking responsibly.

"What to expect and FAQ's" prepares you for the results you will achieve when following the 30-day menu. You will read about how you will feel when you put the menu and the principles in this

book into action. We will also unpack the answers to commonly asked questions about nutrition.

Finally, "*The Weight Loss Equation*" will reveal a simple formula for losing weight. If losing weight is your main objective to be healthier, then you will want to grasp this equation. You might find this information familiar; but understanding the simple formula will help you for a lifetime. This chapter will also ensure your success in preparing for the 30-day menu that is provided for you at the end of the book.

Once you start following the 30-day menu, you will begin to feel **amazing**! That feeling will be your **inspiration** for incorporating whole foods into everyday meals. To guarantee your success, along with the menu, I have provided easy-to-follow recipes and a weekly grocery list.

Changing your habits and living a healthier life can be a long and sometimes difficult journey. Many men and women have traveled this road before you and their stories can often serve as guidelines and encouragement while you take this journey. The stories I have included are about real people, my clients, with real issues regarding their health and weight. I have shared their stories because they deal with common issues most people can relate to. I believe they help to deliver the book's message: to be well, you must eat well.

The Amazing Power of Food
Eat Well. Be Well.

By
Julie Day

Pain of discipline today or the pain of regret tomorrow? You choose.

Steve

Let me tell you a story about my brother-in-law Steve. Steve is a very successful businessman, husband and father of three. He loves his family and tries his best to juggle his family, his job, and his life. At work, he swims in a sea of papers and deadlines. His daily schedule is layered with meetings, appointments, and then school functions and ball games. Steve is trying to survive the proverbial rat race.

Over time, as his children grew older, his financial demands grew and so did his schedule. He began to work harder and longer hours, year after year to move up the corporate ladder, only to wake up and realize how his work had consumed him. He hardly has time for his kids' ball games, much less time to try and eat right and exercise. Steve reminisces about his younger years when he was healthier and life was easier. That was 20 years ago when he weighed 175 pounds and exercised three times a week. He laughs when he tries to imagine feeling that way again. After years of neglecting his health and nutrition, Steve now weighs over 250 pounds. He is on blood pressure and cholesterol medication.

At this point in his life, Steve is very inactive. He has a sedentary job and often eats lunch with clients or grabs lunch on the run. He may dash into the nearest po-boy shop or burger joint just to grab something easy because, as he says, "Who has time to eat well, much less exercise? I need to work and I'm trying to use my time *wisely."*

When Steve finally gets home, he looks for comfort foods. He tells himself he deserves it after the grinding day at work. Exhausted, he pours himself a beer or glass of wine and munches on chips and crackers. Dinner is nothing less than large. Once dinner is over and kids are in bed, it is "Steve" time. He sits back in his favorite chair, watches a little mindless television, which is always accompanied by a snack like popcorn, chocolate, pretzels, or cookies.

While he channel surfs, Steve comes upon the latest fitness infomercial or fad diet commercial and becomes instantly inspired! Just a few minutes of watching and he's hooked! He loves the glitz and glam of the self-made entrepreneur who has made these infomercials and weight loss products. Steve begins to daydream. He begins to think he could be just like those guys on television (tan, muscles, white teeth) if he only had the time. Steve says "I mean, come on, these fitness guys don't work in the 'real' world like I do!" Still, these slick promotions reach their target: he gets inspired! In this moment of inspiration, he buys the latest and greatest health gadget or diet plan, whether it's a shiny new stainless steel juicer that will bring him good health and prosperity in 90 days, or the three-day toxin cleansing pill set that will chisel his abs in 12 days. He rationalizes his purchases as giving him a jumpstart to better health. He needs it--he feels fatigued all day, sleeps poorly, and just loathes himself for allowing himself to become so unhealthy. He believes one of these products will be the solution he has been searching for to get himself into shape.

The juicer arrived on a Friday and so do the cleansing pills. Coincidentally, that evening my husband and I joined Steve and his wife at a food and wine tasting. Knowing my passion for health, Steve excitedly told me about how his new juicer was the jumpstart he needed to bring him better health. "This one is going to work." he said. "I mean, it worked for the guy who lost 90 lbs. in 60 days in the movie, 'I'm Fat, Sick, and Nearly Dead', so why can't it work for me?" I didn't say anything. I just thought about the countless dollars he has spent on the latest fitness trends and on the other dusty machines that haunt his cabinets. Reading my mind he said, "I know what you're thinking, Julie. I know I have purchased things like this before, but they are in the past; they are not a preview into the future." I know his sincerity is there and he really wants to change. I realize that he truly believes this gadget will work and his intentions are genuine and real.

I listened patiently as he explained his newfound healthy ambition and I embraced his desire to want to be healthier. Even though, I so badly wanted to interrupt his juicing story and give him examples of the hundreds of failed "magic pill" attempts and conflictions that I help people recover from every day. I held back. Steve is family, so I tread lightly here.

Then Steve began to explain WHEN he would start his new, wonderful weight loss plan. He couldn't start that week because he had an anniversary dinner to attend the following Tuesday; he justified postponing his new cleansing plan until **after** the anniversary dinner. He felt it was not worth it if he couldn't put one hundred percent into this juicing thing. "It needs to be all or nothing!" Steve exclaimed loudly. He couldn't be more wrong!

I had been quiet up to that point—remember, he is my sister's husband. But when Steve finally got to the part in his justification about "when" he would start this new wonderful weight loss plan, you know, after the anniversary dinner, I couldn't help myself anymore. I blurted out, "Why would you wait 5 days to start any plan? All you have done for the last year is complain about how bad you feel and how tired you are of being overweight. Steve, you have one anniversary meal to "splurge" on out of approximately 15, so why would you wait one more second, much less 5 more days, to finally feel better? That doesn't make any sense at all!" I asked Steve to listen to me for 15 minutes—just give me that. And in those 15 minutes, I highlighted and explained **The Amazing Power of Food** to him. I wanted him to change for a lifetime, but I only asked him for three short days of commitment. I knew if he would just follow these simple guidelines, he would save his life as well as his money. I knew he would feel better and lighter in only three short days. ***I know you can, too.***

Stop over analyzing how you might die and start analyzing how you want to live.

Chapter 1
Inspiration

Where will you find the inspiration to eat well? **Right here**! This book will inspire you to eat well. It will help you stay motivated through your newfound inspiration, so that you can obtain and sustain a healthier body. You are already inspired—you have started to read this book! That means you have already chosen to live a healthier life.

- **Does Inspiration = Motivation?**

--Do you ever feel like you lack motivation to eat better and exercise?

--Do you find that you only try to do better with your exercise and nutrition if some major event is coming up, for example, a vacation or high school reunion, where you feel like all eyes will be evaluating how you look? Are you accountable and determined to eat well when you are not motivated by a big event?

Incentives like these are common and can help you achieve a momentary "fix" regarding your weight. But is that enough? Many people blame "lack of motivation" for their poor eating habits and poor health. The desire to look better, fit into skinny jeans, or wear a bathing suit are decent motivators. However, is motivation what most people lack in regards to their health? I think not. We do not lack *motivation* to be healthier; we lack *inspiration*.

Finding motivation for doing things is easy. For instance, we are motivated to put gas in our car because we know, without it, we cannot go to work. We are motivated to wake up every day because we have responsibilities. *Motivation* seems easy to find.

So what's missing? Inspiration.

Inspiration fuels motivation. Inspiration is a calling to proceed and stay on task even though you may be unsure of your goals or achievements- it may even insist that you go in a direction of uncharted territory. Finding the inspiration to reach your long-term goals and dreams is crucial to your becoming and staying healthy for a lifetime. Eating well to thrive is inspiration. Eating well to feel better for a lifetime is inspiration. Eating well to be the best version of yourself is inspiration. Eating well to live a life full of vitality and strength is inspiration. Search for your own, personal inspiration to be the healthy, strong person you want to be. Inspiration is all around you—just take a look!

- **Finding inspiration**

Do you have children? Someone you care about? Can you find the inspiration to be a role model for them? Ask yourself if you want them to do as you do—they will, you know. Your goals for them should be the same as for yourself--you want them to be as healthy and strong as possible. Learning to eat well can only help you become the best version of yourself and that is a gift you can pass on to your loved ones. By encouraging good eating habits, you can set your children up for a lifetime of success. Imagine how you would feel if you knew for certain that your children would grow up and live healthy, disciplined lives. How would you feel if you knew they had the tools to always manage their weight? That would be a pretty good feeling. They would understand that if they lost self-control and discipline they would live a life full of momentary pleasures and mediocrity. Although life is full of certainty and uncertainty, helping your child or a loved one learn that eating well will lead them to living their "best" life will also inspire *you* to eat well and be the example.

Question: Do you take prescription medication due to a "dis-ease" you may be able to control? Many people from ages forty to seventy take at least two or more daily prescription medications. Think about how many people you know who are taking meds to control cholesterol, blood pressure, thyroid disorders, or diabetes. Taking medicine is not only hard on your body, but wreaks havoc on your pocketbook. If you take control of your own nutrition, you can avoid the need for taking many prescription medications. This fact alone should be inspiration for you to eat well.

You gain inspiration when you inspire others! Do your habits inspire your friends? Changing your habits can certainly inspire friends because when you eat well, and consequently feel better, you become so excited about how good YOU feel that you will want to share it with others. Your inspiration grows when you influence your friends to lead a healthier life. Feeling great is inspiring to others, not to mention infectious. Go beyond eating better to lose a few pounds; eat better to live better and be an inspiration for others!

- **Steps To Stay Inspired**

Staying inspired to eat better can be a challenge, but there are definitely steps you can take that will help you.

--Surround yourself with inspired people who have similar goals

This is the one fact I know to be true. *Who* we are is directly correlated to whom we choose to be around, and quite frankly, we need to be around positive people. Choose carefully the people who surround you on a daily basis. Make sure that these people have the best intentions for your health and wellness. I have seen unhealthy people sabotage others who were trying to lose weight, eat better, or start exercising. This person may be someone in your family or one of your closest friends. Regardless of their relation to you, recognize the people in your life that want you to remain the same and offer resistance, not support, to your healthy changes.

I can say with certainty that if you eat well and start leading a healthier life, you will become more energetic and enthusiastic. Plus, your energy will be contagious! When you gain control over your health, whether you lose weight or just start improving the way you eat, a vitality and exuberance takes over your body. Your enthusiasm will eventually rub off on other people, which may be just what someone else needs to start eating better too.

--Create a positive environment where you live and work

Another way to become more inspired to eat well is by creating a positive environment where you live and work. Keeping inspirational messages close to your desk, or at home, that speak to your heart will help you work toward your goals. Also, you should have a trusted friend or trainer on speed dial to help you if your willpower begins to weaken. Inspiring words from someone you trust and someone who wants to see you achieve your goals can be crucial to your success in leading a healthier lifestyle. My philosophy that people change people, not machines, rings true here. So find that friend or trainer who follows this principle and lean on them when you need inspiration. Staying connected to inspiring people will ensure positive results in your new journey towards good health and wellness. We all need to be reminded of what is possible and achievable.

Remember—you are human. Sometimes you will not feel inspired to eat well. Healthy eating is not always easy, but it is absolutely necessary. Anyone who tells you otherwise is either trying to sell you something or not telling you the truth. No quick fixes, magic pills, special belts, or delicious shakes will melt away the pounds while you sit around and engage in unhealthy habits. Think about it. If losing weight were easy, no one would be struggling to lose those extra inches around his or her waist, and dimpled thighs would disappear. No one would be counting calories or attending spin classes. So accept the challenge and take control of your health. This book contains the tools you need to recapture who you are physically; your journey will be more rewarding than you can ever imagine. I know. I reclaimed my life by making the right (sometimes hard) decisions and committed my life to wellness.

- **Be well AND lose weight**

This book is *not* about losing weight. Losing weight is just one of the side effects of eating well. Do you want to live a lifetime full of vitality and strength? You can unlock your health potential by making smart decisions about food. Being thin or "skinny" does not necessarily translate into being healthy. Everyone knows a "skinny" person who has had a heart attack, lives with diabetes, suffers from depression, or has any number of health-related issues. Fortunately, many of these problems can be prevented, eliminated, or controlled by simply managing what you eat.

Your body needs proper fuel to run efficiently. To perform optimally at work, as a parent, during exercise, or when you are under additional pressure, your body needs the right kind of fuel.

- **Want inspiration? Don't diet!**

Most often, when we attempt to eat healthier, we talk about being on a "diet." The word diet actually means "a temporary change of eating patterns." If a diet is just temporary, then how can it really change you? You will never stay inspired to live on a diet for the rest of your life. To lose weight and keep it off, you have to want to make a fundamental change in your overall health for a lifetime.

--Food-eliminating diets

Many "diet" plans claim to have the secret to weight loss. And yes, some diets help people reach short-term goals, such as wanting to lose ten or fifteen pounds. It is perfectly normal, and

©T h e A m a z i n g P o w e r o f F o o d

helpful, to set goals and work to achieve them. Reaching a goal is satisfying and crucial to the success of any program. But think-- what do you do *after* you have reached that goal? For example, if you lost weight by following a *food eliminating diet* (carb eliminating plans such as Atkins or the Paleo diet) chances are you will have a hard time maintaining that weight loss. People cannot and will not eat "carb-less" for a lifetime. This kind of diet does not last and neither do the results. Why? Meals that contain carbohydrates, red meat, and a glass of wine, for instance, all taste very good and have a place in a healthy lifestyle. Losing weight by eliminating food groups gives you a narrow margin for long-term success in maintaining your health and weight loss goals. When weight loss is no longer your only motivator to eat better, you will see change in your health and weight.

--*Beware of foods that masquerade as healthy, diet foods*

Again, when weight loss is strictly your motivation, it is likely that you will reach out to the pre-packaged, quick-fix meals or snacks that tend to fool you, the consumer. Commercials promise us that foods like 100-calorie snack packs or frozen dinners will be healthy alternatives in our diet but, in fact, they are quite the opposite. Take a look in the frozen food section of the grocery store. Here you will find "low-calorie" frozen dinners and low calorie desserts—meals packaged and ready for you to prepare quickly after a long day at work. Unfortunately, most of these prepared meals are loaded with sodium and other unhealthy additives—just read the labels. The list of chemicals added to your food is frightening—you have no idea what you are putting in your body; you just know it's only 350 calories—but of what?

The food industry has conveniently packaged snacks and desserts into "small" 100-calorie packs of processed delight. These products (or clever marketing) convince us that this food-like product will help us overcome the bulge and be easy on our budget. WRONG! These snacks are nothing more than 100 calories. They are void of any nutritional value. That 100-calorie snack will just stir your appetite and leave you hungry. I have yet to meet anyone who eats only one package of these treats. *"If it's only 100 calories then I can afford two!"* is the usual mentality.

--Real, whole food

Incorporating real, whole foods into your meals and snacks is the only way to reclaim your health and live a life full of energy. We can either fuel our bodies to be healthy or unhealthy. Those are the only two options. Making the right food choices is not always easy, but making better decisions about the food you eat will lead to a healthier life. Whether you need to lose over 100 pounds or you just want to feel better, the *Amazing Power Of Food* will teach you HOW to make better decisions when it comes time to eat, which will fuel your life-long inspiring journey of being healthy.

- **Take a risk for your health!**

Break the chains of conformity! Stop your old way of doing things. Take a risk for your health—you have nothing to lose but poor health and a new life full of vitality to gain. Make a commitment to healthier eating and disregard that lazy attitude toward preparing the food you eat.

Being healthy doesn't have to be complicated! Right here you will receive simple education, simple recipes, menus and guidelines to help you choose wisely. I believe you have a life or death choice before you today: you can choose to eat unhealthy foods that bring about poor nutrient levels and degeneration which accelerates your aging process; OR you can choose to eat real whole foods that help protect you from disease and aging and bring you more energy.

There are three things you must KNOW and truly BELIEVE to be successful with your health and weight:

- You *can* be healthy!
- You *can* be at the weight you desire no matter your age!
- You *can* feel better than ever before!

The following chapters and menus provided in this book can certainly help solve all confusion about nutrition and help anyone acquire a healthy life. By practicing a few simple guidelines, which are outlined in the upcoming chapters, you can become stronger, healthier, wiser, smarter, and more disease-resistant. Change your lifestyle through education of WHY certain foods are better than others.

It is not hard to live a healthy lifestyle. It just takes a little preparation, discipline, and a new mindset about your body. Food is the key to good health and the driving force behind being healthy. Nutrition, good or bad, affects everything you do and the level at which you are able to do it.

Do what it takes to remain inspired because you are closer than you think to a healthier body and to becoming the best version of yourself. No more worries about dieting. Eating foods that are more nutrient dense can lead to weight loss. And what does weight loss lead to? Studies show that losing 10-15% of your body weight decreases medical problems and improves heart function, blood pressure, cholesterol levels, lipid profiles, glucose tolerance and sleep disorders. It can also decrease medication requirements, duration of hospitalizations, and post-operative complications.

Why wait? Your new, more energetic life begins now! Sickness and disease is the body's way of telling you it's time to do things differently. Take control of your body by changing the foods you eat, and watch illness and low energy fade away.

Suggestions on becoming and remaining inspired

- ❖ *Surround yourself with the right people.*
- ❖ *Do not be afraid to call on someone's help.*
- ❖ *Read books or articles that support the importance of eating well.*
- ❖ *Eat well to be well, not just to lose weight.*
- ❖ *Remind yourself eating well is not always easy but necessary.*
- ❖ *Do not become discouraged with slip-ups.*
- ❖ *Act as role model for someone you care about.*
- ❖ *Try to inspire friends and family to join you in the quest of living a healthier life.*

Eating the right thing when you feel like eating the wrong thing is called progress.

Chapter 2

What do you really want?

As a fitness professional, I meet with clients one-on-one to discuss how to begin a successful nutrition program. During these meetings, the first question I ask is **"What do you want out of these nutrition sessions? Really, it doesn't matter if it sounds like it may be impossible...tell me, what do you want?"** Some clients tell me things like "I want to lose weight" or "I want to fit in my old jeans" or "I just want to feel better." They begin to talk about the real results they want regarding their health and weight and when I tell them it's completely possible to get those results (because it is always possible as long as we endure a little discipline and hard work) the battle is half over. So, the first step in becoming healthier is to take a few minutes and answer the following question. Write down three things you really want regarding your overall wellness. This is a crucial step to getting the results you want. Don't limit yourself.

What do you want?

1. _Amy - More energy_

2. _Amy - Better mental sharpness_

3. _Amy - loose 15 lbs_

The second step to better health is to analyze your daily routine regarding the food you eat. I ask my clients many questions about their daily nutrition habits; these questions really open their eyes. At first they're a bit hesitant to be honest about what they eat; they do not want to be criticized or judged. But once they begin to open up, either by telling me or writing down their response, something powerful and enlightening occurs. They come face to face with their own eating behavior. Through this process they become more mindful of their actions and behaviors, an important step that we cannot overlook as we begin the process of becoming healthier.

Here are specific questions for you to answer that will help you recognize your own daily routine. Your answers will allow you to see the food choices you tend to make every day. Be honest with yourself: write down the good, the bad, and the ugly. If you have been trying to eat better for two weeks, do not list those choices. Recall how you have been eating for the past several years: write down *that* information. It is in your best interest to recall what you do on a daily basis; fully admit your food weaknesses and strengths.

MORNING

1. What time do you wake up every morning?

   Amy- 6:45 Am

2. What is the first thing you do after waking up most mornings? (For example, take a shower, brush your teeth, drink a cup of coffee...)

   Amy- go to the bathroom

3. If you eat breakfast, what do you like to eat?

   Amy-Don't eat breakfast- Have a protein shake

4. What do you typically eat for breakfast?

   Amy - Protein Shake

5. Do you ever snack between breakfast and lunch? If so, what do you snack on most days?

   Amy-Yes- granola bar, nuts or yogurt

6. Do you drink any beverages in the morning? (For example, diet drinks, coffee, water, etc.)

   Amy Spark - energy/vitamin Drink

© T h e A m a z i n g P o w e r o f F o o d

LUNCH & AFTERNOON

7. What do you like to eat for lunch?

Amy- Soup, left overs, take out

8. What do you typically eat for lunch? Be very specific. Remember to write down what you eat on days you feel you are eating well or poorly.

Amy- Frozen meal, Chinese, sandwich, ChickFilA, Bojangles

9. Do you ever have a sweet snack after lunch? If so, what do you typically choose? Would you eat it immediately after lunch or an hour or so later?

Amy - yes; Chocolate (bite size); a couple hours after lunch

10. Do you ever snack between lunch and dinner? If so, what do you most often choose to eat?

Amy- Chocalate (bite size), mixed nuts, granola bar

DINNER AND AFTER

11. What time do you eat dinner? (Between 4-6pm, 5-7pm, 6-8pm or later?)

Between 5-7 pm

©The Amazing Power of Food

12. What do you most often eat for dinner?

Amy - Fish, chicken, w/rice, potatoes, veggies Tacos, eggs + toast

13. Do you ever snack after dinner? List all possible snacks you may eat.

Amy - yes; granola bar, mixed nuts, Chocolate or cookies if we have them.

14. What time do you go to bed most nights?

Amy - between 10:30-11:30 pm

OTHER INFORMATION

15. How much water do you drink per day?

Amy - At least 1/2 gallon

16. Do you take vitamins? If so, please list all vitamins. *Yes- multi, omega's, calcium, iron*

17. Do you drink alcohol? If so, how often and what is your beverage of choice? *Yes- 4-6 drinks per year*

© T h e   A m a z i n g   P o w e r   o f   F o o d

Now go back and read over all of your answers and take a look at how you fuel your body. Do you eat meals? Are your days filled with mostly whole foods, fruits, and vegetables? Are your days filled with mostly processed convenient fast food? What commonality do you find in all of your meals? Would you want someone you love or someone you care about to follow the diet you have just described? Are you proud of the food choices you make every day? Is there room for improvement? Is there one specific time every day that your lose control and regret what you eat? For instance, you eat a good breakfast and a fairly decent lunch, but by three in the afternnon you need a boost and will eat anything and everything. By answering these questions honestly and analyzing how and what you eat, you will see where you need to make improvements with your nutrition.

Writing down your habitual food choices allows you to see just how much thought, or lack thereof, you put into your meals every day. It is important to point out that poor eating habits that weaken you are relatively easy and result from acting mindlessly, while eating habits that allow you to be your best require thought, effort, and discipline.

The next step is to learn how to eat well. The information you find in the next chapter should make sense and not confuse you. Get ready for a new mindset! Be excited—you are on your way to accomplish what you really want - a healthier version of you!

Suggestions for accomplishing what you really want

❖ *Be honest with yourself about what and when you eat.*

❖ *Find the time of day that you are most challenged.*

❖ *Fill that weak time with activities to divert your attention, such as a walk or a trip to the gym.*

❖ *Learn how to snack wisely to boost your nutrition and energy.*

❖ *Know you are not alone in having "bad" days or "weak" moments.*

❖ *Let go of fad diets that may have worked in the past.*

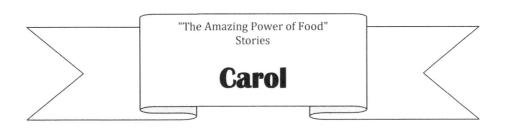

"Julie, I've got to talk to you! Do you have a minute?" Even though I was training a client, I was eager to know what was on her mind. She pulled me aside and told me about a weight loss consultation she had experienced the night before. She began by telling me it was a free diet consultation sponsored by the local hospital where she works. They were promoting a popular, multi-level marketing diet and I could tell by her expression that her consultation experience was less than she had hoped; I had a feeling her story would be one I had heard many times before. Since Carol wanted extreme results, extremely quickly, she thought this new extreme diet would be exactly the thing she needed to lose 50 pounds in a couple of months. It would be the "kick start" to a new, healthier Carol.

She described how excited she was when she arrived at her consultation only to be immediately taken back by the age of her consultation representative--she looked no older than 15. "I thought she looked very young and inexperienced." Carol said. Nonetheless, she was willing to hear what the young woman had to say.

To begin, the representative never asked Carol any questions regarding her health or physical condition. Instead she immediately started describing the diet. "On this diet plan you can eat as much lettuce as you want, you can expect to feel really bad for at least two weeks, and you can NOT exercise while on this plan." Then the representative pulled out several bottles of expensive supplements that Carol would have to purchase if she decided to do the diet. She was told that since she couldn't get her nutrients from food, she would have to get them in pill form. Carol thanked her and left empty-handed.

Who in their right mind wants to feel bad, not move for weeks and starve--not me or anyone else I know. But if your local hospital or workplace promotes this type of plan, you can see how people could be seduced by this flash-in-the-pan diet. Unfortunately, people do fall for the "quick fix" very often, only to have it result in failure. The food that nature provides for us has all the nutrients we need, so why should we try to supplement our bodies with man-made pills? Supplements can never give us the disease-fighting properties that whole foods contain.

Chapter 3
Keeping Food Choices Simple

- **And No More Diets!**

No need to feel overwhelmed by the multitude of diet plans and diet books; don't worry about choosing which of the following is right for you: the 3-Day Diet, Cabbage Soup Diet, Atkins Diet, South Beach Diet, 17-Day Diet, Eat Right For Your Blood Type Diet, Tapeworm Diet (yes, this is a real diet with real tapeworms), and The Paleo Diet, just to name a few. Many of these short-term programs promise rapid weight loss, but they do not work long term. Many of these fad diets lack carbohydrates, leading to muscle and liver glycogen depletion. Since water is stored with carbohydrates, when you stop eating carbohydrates you will notice a rapid water-weight loss. But guess what? Water weight always returns! When that happens, your resolve melts away instead of your pounds.

Confusion abounds concerning the multitude of diet plans that are out there but confusion is not necessary. There is an easier way of understanding your body and weight loss.

- **To lose weight—simply eat fewer calories than you burn!**

Losing weight is as simple as it is difficult. Just remember, to lose weight you have to eat fewer calories than you burn. All we have to do is some basic math, yet we continue to try to search for more complicated ways to accomplish our goals. Using portion control, paying attention to that simple equation mentioned above (*eating less, doing more),* and eating more whole foods will provide you with good health and permanent weight loss. Don't convolute this process.

- **Read labels carefully: what "light" "fat-free" "reduced" and "sugar-free" really mean**

  A diet based in whole foods such as apples, carrots, broccoli, spinach and kale are what we need to eat to be healthier. However, when people try to eat better, with weight loss as a primary goal, they often turn to foods and products that claim to be fat-free, light, reduced, sugar-free, etc. Often these foods are worse for us nutritionally. Read the labels carefully. Avoid buying products loaded with artificial flavors and sweeteners just to spare a few calories. Here are a few common terms found on packaged foods. If you understand what these terms mean, you will choose foods more wisely.

  Light: (1) a nutritionally-altered product that contains 1/3 fewer calories or 1/2 of the fat of the referenced food; (2) a low-calorie, low-fat food whose sodium content has been reduced by 50%. If a food product contains the word "*light*" on the packaging, it often indicates the product was sweetened with artificial sweeteners.

  Reduced: This food (whether altered or not) contains 25% less of a nutrient or calories than the reference food (for example, "reduced-fat" milk, or "reduced-sodium" soup). "Fewer" is an acceptable synonym.

Healthy: A healthy food must be low in fat and saturated fat and contain limited amounts of sodium and cholesterol per serving. Examples include "heart-healthy" soups or cereals.

Free: This term means that a product contains none or only a trivial amount of a food component. Examples include "fat-free" ice-cream, milk, etc.

Low: This term, expressed in "per serving" amounts, can be used on foods that can be eaten frequently without exceeding dietary guidelines (fat: 3 grams or less, saturated fat: 1 gram or less, cholesterol: 20g or less, sodium: 35 mg or less, and calories: 40 kcal or less per serving). Examples include low-sodium chicken broth or low-fat yogurt.

- **Whole foods are the key to successful eating**

  Eating well is really so simple—just concentrate on eating real, whole foods (fruits, vegetables, beans, lentils, nuts, seeds and whole grains) everyday and with every meal. You do not need to complicate your life with elaborate recipes or fake foods. Nor must you cook all the time to eat better. The cleaner you eat, the less cooking is necessary. Cooking your food to death will not give you the vital nutrients you need. Food loses fiber, vitamins, and minerals when cooked over 118 degrees. Further, overcooking meat and vegetables can oxidize and destroy heat-susceptible vitamins, such as the B group, C and E. Boiling vegetables leaches out the water-soluble B group and C, as well as many minerals.

Also, some vitamins, such as B6, can be destroyed by microwaving. You don't always have to eat raw food, but understand that fresh fruits and fresh (or lightly steamed) vegetables IS the healthy choice.

Fresh fruits are considered whole foods. I have noticed that people have an easier time eating fresh fruit earlier in the day. Incorporating fresh fruit in your breakfast or mid -morning snack provides essential vitamins you need to be healthy. If fresh produce is in your line of vision you will be more likely to eat it. So leave fresh fruit out on your countertop, or place it in a clear container in your refrigerator where you can see it. You may eat more of these foods if you just keep them within sight.

Adding whole foods to every meal can be as simple as eating fresh carrots with your sandwich at lunch or loading your sandwiches with fresh vegetables. Try to eat fresh or lightly steamed vegetables with dinner. Lightly steaming vegetables only takes about five minutes and they are loaded with vitamins. Also, have a salad for a meal once a day. This will ensure a calorie deficit and a nutrient surplus. Having whole foods *available* is usually the biggest hurdle to overcome. So go to the store once a week to purchase fresh food and make the food easily accessible.

- **Restaurants 101**

So many of us come home after a long day, overworked, and too tired to think about cooking a meal. For many, dining out 2-3 times a day in fast-food chains or restaurants has become a way of life. Studies have shown that dining out all the time is the real culprit behind our country's enormous obesity rate: **You have no control over the sodium, fat, calories, or additives in foods that you do not prepare.**

I suggest you prepare and eat more of your own meals if you really want to be healthier and lose weight. When you are in control of your food, you are in better control of your physical health. Leaving your health in the hands of fast-food chains and most restaurants can be risky. Does that mean that you can't eat out without feeling guilty? Not at all. Begin to view dining out as a luxury. It should be a wonderful experience that can be fun, relaxing, and tasty. If you choose to dine out only once or twice a week, do not worry about the caloric consequence. Rather, focus on your other weekly meals to make a greater impact on your health and weight. For instance, if you eat well and prepare your own meals Sunday through Friday, and you choose to go out to dinner Friday or Saturday night, enjoy your meals on those nights. You earned it!

On the other hand, if eating out often is your way of life, and you have chosen not to change your lifestyle, then you need to pay close attention to what and how you eat. The same whole food principle applies here: every meal eaten "out" should contain *whole foods*.

Perhaps your family frequents a Mexican restaurant because it is inexpensive and the food tastes good. You want to eat well and you are determined to stay on course. If this is the case,

© T h e   A m a z i n g   P o w e r   o f   F o o d

then I suggest you order fresh foods with your meal. Fresh choices at a Mexican restaurant are foods like Pico de gallo (fresh tomatoes, jalapenos, and onions), steamed vegetables, and grilled chicken fajitas. This meal acts as a healthy alternative to foods such as cheese enchiladas or beef burritos loaded with a day's worth of sodium and fat. Incorporating fresh, whole foods with your meals is simple and can be used at any restaurant. Almost every restaurant offers fresh salads and other fresh foods; consider asking for a grilled or steamed alternative to something fried. If the item does not appear on the menu, you may have to ask your server; usually the restaurant will be able to accommodate you.

In short, if you limit eating out to only a couple of meals a week, then by all means enjoy yourself when you get the chance to have a great dining experience. You should look forward to having someone wait on you and prepare your food. Relax and enjoy the meal. Choose healthy alternatives when you can. If not, enjoy your little splurge and do not feel guilty. But if your goal is to lose weight, control your cholesterol, lower your blood pressure, and just be healthier, then limit eating out and prepare your own meals throughout the week. Remember, your goal is to stay on track with your sodium, fat, and food additives.

Suggestions for keeping it simple

❖ *When in doubt stick to real, whole foods not packaged.*

❖ *Every meal should contain something "real."*

❖ *Do not cook your food to death, literally.*

❖ *Watch out for fad & food-eliminating diets; they end in failure.*

❖ *Avoid eating manipulated foods, such as sugar-free, light, and some fat-free products.*

❖ *Stop smoking! Smoking causes depletion of vitamin C to the tune of 25 to 100 milligrams per cigarette.*

Chapter 4
Identify Your Eating Patterns

How you eat is just as important as what you eat. Let me explain. In my years of helping people redefine their health, I have discovered crucial mistakes people make regarding the *way* they eat. Some people never get around to eating until early or mid-afternoon—these are the back-loaders. Some people never actually sit down and eat a full meal, but nibble all day long—these are the grazers. Both back-loading and grazing are dangerous eating behaviors that can lead to poor health and weight gain.

- **Back-loaders**

Back-loaders consume all of their calories at the end of the day. Back-loading calories like this is extremely detrimental to your well-being causing fatigue, poor health, and weight gain.

Back-loaders usually skip breakfast. When a person habitually skips breakfast, it is usually because they ate too many calories snacking the night before. That caloric damage makes people feel like they don't deserve to eat the next morning. Eating late night snacks, such as ice cream, salty chips, popcorn, or chocolate (you know, the "fun" snacks we like to eat while watching television or a good movie) can affect your blood sugar, cause night sweats, and usually disrupt sleep. Interrupted sleep patterns make waking up the next morning an enormous challenge.

Mindless night-time snacking can easily add up to approximately 400 calories (or more) before bedtime and often results in dehydration and of course, weight gain. Since breakfast has been skipped, typically a diet drink or coffee helps to fight off mid-morning hunger pangs. Even though water would be the best choice at this time of day, it won't satisfy this kind of eater; at this point, a jolt is all they need (or it's what they *think* they need).

By lunchtime, the back-loader has not eaten anything of any substantial nutrition nor consumed many calories of any kind. Now they feel absolutely starved! This overwhelming sense of starvation leads to poor food choices. Even the *most* disciplined people find it nearly impossible to make healthy choices when they are starving. Back-loaders, now look for the quick lunch fix because their bodies are crying for fuel! Frequently, a drive-thru or any other fast-food alternative, jammed full of processed meats, trans fats, sodium, and hydrogenated oils, immediately calms the starving body. After lunch, a vicious craving for something sweet kicks in. No meal is complete without that sweet treat to punctuate a thoroughly unhealthy meal decision. It may be a few chocolate morsels or a trip to the vending machine at work, but living without that treat makes life unbearable for this kind of eater. Back-loaders rationalize and justify their poor food choices, assuming they can afford the calories since they skipped breakfast—a huge misconception.

Anyone who skips meals and is "starving" will usually eat too many calories at one given time. The human body has a hard time trying to digest and eliminate hundreds (or thousands) of calories eaten all at once. This isn't hard to do when convenient, fast-food is the easy choice. Your body cannot handle distributing that many calories, that much fat, or sodium at one time. If fast-food is something you eat often, then I suggest you read a fast-food nutrition chart that you can find on the internet. I recommend reviewing *www.fastfoodnutrition.org*. Look up the nutrition facts regarding your favorite fast-food meals. I guarantee you will be shocked at what you find.

Here are just a few stats you may find interesting:

1. On average, a fast-food "meal deal" contains over 1500-2000 calories.

2. Only *one* slice of delivery cheese pizza has over 300 calories and approximately 600-800 milligrams of sodium.

3. Classic fast-food chicken sandwiches have over 400 calories, a whopping 1,400 milligrams of sodium, and nearly 20 grams of fat--that doesn't include french fries or a drink.

Back-loaders are usually the consummate yo-yo dieters. These eaters generally conform to the *all-or-nothing* approach about eating well. They actually think about eating healthy, but choose not to out of habit. Quite simply they starve themselves too long and then always rush to eat poor food choices.

Because back-loaders have not given their body any proper "fuel," they will feel ridiculously hungry again come mid-afternoon or early evening. This is a dangerous time; now they reach for the "grab-able" food, or what I call "edible" products. There is a big difference between *real food* and *edible* products. Edible products are things like crackers, pretzels, granola bars, protein bars, hard candies, candy bars, chips and gummy candies just to name a few. You can eat these products and not suffer any immediate side effects, however, edible products provide relatively little to no nutritional value--just a handful of empty calories.

When dinnertime arrives, a quick, thoughtless meal will more than likely suffice for this kind of eater. Since back-loaders feel chronically fatigued from not properly fueling their body all day long, they are exhausted by early evening. They have no energy to prepare a meal. High calories + high fat + low nutrient levels = **fatigue**. Due to poor lunch choices and hectic schedules, back-loaders have to overcome their lack of motivation to even consider making a healthy dinner. Thus the cycle repeats itself relying on fast-food or frozen, already-prepared food for their meals. So dinner is another meal delivered quickly and conveniently, but offering no other benefits. For some, the meal is accompanied with a glass or two of wine and of course, a sweet treat to follow. From morning till night, poor decisions are being made. Can you relate to this type of eater? Do you fall into this eating category? If not, maybe you fall into the second most popular eating category.

- **Grazers**

As the name implies, this type of eater likes to graze on food throughout the day. Grazing is another detrimental eating behavior that contributes to poor health, fatigue, and weight gain.

In the morning grazers often take a quick bite from their

kids' breakfast plates or snack on a few bites of dinner leftovers. Throughout the morning grazers munch on foods, such as cold pizza, a turkey roll up, or a few handfuls of dry cereal. Every hour or so they may snack on a handful of nuts, processed granola bar, or anything that doesn't resemble a meal. Grazers often rationalize their food choices because they think they are only eating a mouthful of food at a time. Somehow those calories don't count; they might not even remember eating them. Just like any other food you eat, calories from these mouthfuls cannot be ignored. Nutritional values and calories absolutely count. Because constant oral stimulation seems to be a part of this eating personality, grazers will typically have a diet drink, regular soft drink, or maybe an ice tea nearby; they constantly ingest useless fuel (not to mention extraordinarily unhealthy fuel) into their body.

People who fall into this category find it common practice to eat alone and most often stand up while eating. They don't feel comfortable eating around others and would rather not engage in a dining experience.

Grazing constantly throughout the day has many negative side effects. Grazers eat mostly easy-to-grab, processed carbohydrates without realizing how much they are actually eating. They don't get the appropriate amount of nutrients they need to feel satisfied or sustain healthy living. They get calories, not nutrients. This way of eating generally results in very low fiber intake, which can cause an insatiable appetite.

Though these two eating personalities are not the only two

types of unhealthy eaters to be sure, many people, frustrated with their eating patterns, fall into one of these categories. You may recognize one of these as your own, just not quite as extreme. Or you may eat a bit differently. Either way, it is important for everyone to recognize their own eating habits and implement the changes necessary to live and *maintain* a healthy lifestyle.

Some suggestions to identify how you eat

- ❖ *Keep a food log for one week.*
- ❖ *Analyze your food log, review the time of your meals and add up the caloric intake.*
- ❖ *Recognize the time of the day that you may eat poorly and prepare for it ahead of time.*

Chapter 5
Eliminate Excuses

- **Choose wisely: Do what you *know*, not what you *feel***

No matter how you have been eating or what your daily routine may be, the good news is that it is relatively easy to implement new behaviors to correct poor eating habits. In order for you to be healthier you MUST make changes if you want your future to look different from your past. Your life will change when your habits change.

To ensure nutritional success, do away with excuses for eating poorly and being less of what you were made to be. Everyone is presented with a *choice* of food at meal times and making the right choice is crucial to your health. Ask yourself this question: Which *choice* will help you become your "best" self? Coming home from work and sitting on the couch with a bag of chips and a beer or going for a brisk walk or run? The answer is easy. Every food situation can be approached with this question but first you must do away excuses for making bad choices.

Excuse #1: "I'm an emotional eater."

I can safely say that seventy percent of the clients whom I coach nutritionally define themselves as emotional eaters. Emotional eating becomes their number one excuse behind making bad food choices. They have used this excuse for years for not being able to control their health and their weight. We all have emotions—we feel at any given time happy, sad, confused, flabbergasted, or whatever. We are emotional everyday of our lives and will be for the rest of lives, so how can the excuse of eating because you are emotional be valid? If you define yourself as an "emotional" eater then it is even more important for you to manage your emotions; do not allow them to manage you. When you emotionally eat you often eat things that you think will make you happy, only to discover that what you ate ends up making you miserable. Often people confuse pleasure with happiness. Sometimes long-term misery comes conveniently disguised as short-term pleasure.

Making emotional wellness a priority will help you in every area of your life, and this includes making healthy decisions about what you eat. Emotions can urge you towards the "quick fix"; then you suffer the guilt afterwards. The cycle perpetuates more emotion. You feel guilty about what you've eaten and what do you do next? You eat! Riding an emotional rollercoaster and having food involved in the process leaves you exhausted and emotionally drained. When you gluttonously overeat under the veil of emotional eating you are left in despair and full of self-loathing. This is not a healthy place to be and we find ourselves there simply by having made poor food choices when it came time to eat.

Leading a healthier life through nutrition will allow you to become stable, solid, steadfast, and determined no matter what emotional state you are in. Allowing your emotions to control you, your health, and the decisions you make will never give you positive results. However, there is an easy fix. Try making nutritional decisions according to what you *know,* not what you *feel.* What DO you know? You know you must eat well to feel well.

Excuse #2: "I just don't have time to eat well!"

Another common excuse for not eating well is that people can't find the *time* to eat well. They are too busy. Their busy lifestyle does not allow any extra time for them to think ahead and prepare things to eat. Do any of the following scenarios sound familiar?

--you work through lunch so you can pick up your children an hour earlier from daycare.

--you use your lunch break to run errands.

--too busy to eat breakfast and lunch, you graze instead; by three in the afternoon you desperately swing by a drive-thru and grab yourself (and maybe your kids) a quick, convenient "snack" before ball practice, dance, or just another set of errands.

--you spend your lunch hour having "business lunches" which possibly add more stress rather than more good fuel to your system.

--your grocery cart is full of "prepared" foods—edible, easy-to-grab, processed meals and snacks because you think you have no time, nor energy to focus on anything else.

Unfortunately, for many people these scenarios play out daily. People continually claim their busy schedule is the culprit behind their poor health. However, at the end of the day, you must take full responsibility for your schedule. **Be aware:** *If your life is* *so busy that it does not allow time for something as fundamental to your well-being as eating, then there is something inherently wrong with your time management skills.*

With a minimal amount of preparation and planning, you can have meals and snacks lined up that are easy, fast, tasty, and most importantly, healthy. How busy you are, is not an excuse to eat poorly; you may just need to manage your time better. Begin to take responsibility for how you eat and how you are going to prepare healthier food. No more excuses! **Excuses guarantee failure because you have accepted failure as a possibility.**

- **Self-control: Practice makes Perfect**

You will feel fully alive when you embrace a life of discipline and self-control in regards to eating. Discipline is an essential element in becoming healthy and happy. If you want to measure your happiness, try measuring your discipline--these two are directly correlated to one another. Being disciplined (and thus having self-control) is the key to freedom--freedom from the bondage and burdens that being overweight and unhealthy can cause. Freedom is being able to play with your kids or grandkids. Freedom is being able to climb a flight of stairs with ease. Freedom is being able to live free from medication and weekly doctor visits. Discipline will never enslave or stifle you, but rather set you free to reach unimaginable heights. Human beings thrive on discipline. Are you thriving or just surviving? Practicing discipline and self-control are critical to your success in changing the way you eat and the food choices you make. Self-control does not just happen; it needs to be developed and practiced. We develop self-control by using it, just as we can develop muscles by using them. The more we practice, the easier it is to make better decisions.

Self-control and respect for your body go hand in hand. The body you have been given is the *only* body you will EVER have. Respect it! Your body has a big job to do, and you are the only one who can help. Eating well will get you where you need to be in life. When you do not practice self-control in what you choose to eat, you show a lack of respect for your body. When you lack respect for your body, you live in regret. When you live in regret, you live with low self-esteem. When you live with low self- esteem, you don't enjoy life. Whew! Jump off this vicious carousel now! Start respecting yourself more by eating well, and watch your health and your life improve each and every day!

Ninety-nine percent of the time you are in control of what your body becomes. Healthy bodies are created little by little over days, weeks, months, and years through thousands of seemingly insignificant acts of self-control and discipline. It is not too late to reclaim your health. Even if you feel like too much damage has already been done, it hasn't. You have amazing control over your cellular body AND genetics for that matter.

Think of your genetics wired with a light switch that you turn on and off. Most of what happens to your physical body is not determined by your genetics. You choose whether or not you allow your genetics to control your future. That's right, you choose! For example, just because your mother, father, or both have type 2 diabetes does not mean that you will automatically inherit the same disease. Type 2 diabetes is an environmental disease. It is self-induced by abusing your body year after year. Living sedentary lifestyles, having poor eating habits, and drinking too much alcohol all promote this disease. You cannot keep making excuses for eating too much and moving too little. Make the decision now to have more self-control and be in charge of your life! Respect yourself! Give yourself the gift of good health by acquiring the discipline to eat well.

Edit that lazy attitude right out of your brain. Don't listen to the voice that says, "I don't have time to stop at the grocery store to buy some fruit and veggies—I'll just stop this one time at the drive-thru, so I can have more time to....". Living life to the fullest takes effort and discipline.

Through my personal experience of working with many people, I have sadly discovered that self-discipline is almost non-existent and our society is becoming more ill because of its absence. Therefore, practice self-discipline a work toward making it a priority. Become a role model for your family, your children, and those around you. By becoming more self-disciplined, you will make better decisions about what you eat. Through discipline, you will have healthy foods readily available, and eating well becomes much easier.

Living in good health does not happen by accident. Good health is always **practiced and planned**. Ask anyone who is in good health, and you will find that they practice healthy habits—they aren't lucky. Practice can be defined as "*a repeated performance of systematic exercise for the purpose of acquiring skill or proficiency.*" The more you practice the discipline of being prepared, the more you plan your meals, the more proficient you will become, and the less time it will take. Practice makes perfect—or at least makes life much easier.

Suggestions for eliminating excuses

❖ *Accept the fact that there is no excuse for being unhealthy.*

❖ *Separate emotions and food as much as possible. You live with emotions, and you need food to live. These two things must not influence each other in a negative way.*

❖ *There are 168 hours in a week. It takes 1 hour a week to go to the store and pick up healthy food choices. You have the time; you just have to use it wisely.*

Veronica

Veronica is a strong and beautiful 32-year old woman who is about 50 pounds overweight. She has attempted to lose weight many different ways: counting calories, fasting, and cutting out all carbohydrates. She tried Weight Watchers, The Atkins Diet, The South Beach Diet, and The Paleo Diet. With each attempt she would typically lose about 10 pounds in the first two weeks. After those two weeks she found that counting all of those calories just became too hard, fasting made her too tired, and/or carbohydrates just tasted too good to give up. All of her attempts to lose weight and keep it off failed.

Frustrated, but once again determined, Veronica was ready for a change. She realized she was too young to feel so tired, unhealthy, and out of control. She was depressed about how she felt and looked. Plus, she wanted to be a good example for her 10-year old daughter who was also overweight. Veronica came to me desperately looking for help.

As she began to talk about her eating habits, I realized her basic notions about food plans were misguided. She believed that if she ate one "bad" thing, she had blown any chance to recover. Immediately, she became disappointed in herself, proceeded to self-sabotage and ate terribly until the next diet phase came along. This behavior is known as "yo-yo" dieting, a vicious cycle of starting to lose weight, stopping the program, then gaining all the lost weight back. It is what I call the "all or nothing" approach--it will **never, ever** work!

As I analyzed what Veronica ate every day, I shared with her the dangers of what this "yo-yo" dieting abuse was doing to her health. I forecasted what her health would look like in ten years if she kept this vicious cycle going. If she continued on this path, in ten years she would gain even more weight and possibly become a diabetic. With the extra weight she would eventually gain, she would become even more inactive, which in turn would lead to numerous other poor health conditions.

Veronica is a passionate woman who really appreciates good food--she is what I call a "foodie". She loves watching the Food Network, intrigued by challenging recipes, new restaurants, and promising chefs. But she really hadn't gained much knowledge about what she should eat to be healthy.

During our sessions she learned the importance of eating whole foods and how powerful they can be. Inspired, when she went to the local grocery store she filled her basket full of fresh produce to make her own healthy, homemade meals. Encouraged by the simple recipes I gave her, she had no trouble cooking healthy. Plus, she realized how much she enjoyed preparing and cooking with fresh whole foods. She just had never taken the time or made the effort to buy those foods before we met. Once she realized how invaluable certain foods were to her declining health, she found that preparing *her own meals was worth the effort. Veronica is now close to her goal weight, and she continues to eat more whole foods than ever before. Not only does she feel better, she sees the change in her daughter as well—they both have lost weight, slowly but steadily, and have become more active. Now she knows that even though she ate her way into poor health, she can also eat her way out of it.*

Chapter 6
Untie Your Food

- **If You Fall...Get Back Up**

Do you resemble Veronica? Do you have an all or nothing attitude about eating food? See if you recognize yourself in the following scenarios: You went to the movies, ate too much popcorn and way too many M&M's. When you got home and saw that last piece of cake sitting on the counter, you figure you might as well just eat that too. Or, you just attended an event, e.g., a birthday party, wedding, or dinner party where sugar plum fairies created irresistible treats, and you did not resist. You indulged. You chock it up to having a bad day and decide to polish off a bag of Oreos as soon as you get home.

We mess up! It's understandable that sometimes a piece of cheesecake (or insert your favorite food here) will stalk you and force you to eat it. It happens to everyone; no one eats well **all** of the time. An occasional sweet treat or caloric splurge is truly not that big of a deal as long as the splurge stops right there. To ensure a lifetime of success of healthy eating, **untie your food**.

Tying bad food choices together, for instance, "blowing it" at lunch and continuing to "blow it" the rest of the day or weekend is dangerous. Untie your food and make up for that bad meal at the next mealtime. If you indulge and have a big, not so healthy lunch and really overeat, your next meal needs to be lower in calories and nutrient rich.

Everyone eats too much at times. It's just a part of human nature, especially nowadays when food is so readily available. Think of your food mishaps as you would babies learning how to walk. When babies learn how to walk, they always fall. And every time a baby falls, they don't just sit on the floor feeling sorry for themselves. They get back up and keep trying. They may bump their head or skin their knees, but they *will* walk.

When you are choosing to eat your way into a better lifestyle by eating healthier, more nutritious meals, you will encounter a day (or meal) of poor eating every now and then. You will fall. It's going to happen. But don't give up by letting one bad meal roll into the next. Just like a baby learning how to walk, when you fall down, get back up and be as consistent as possible in making healthier food choices. If you have one "bad" meal, eat better at your next meal and choose healthier foods.

When you continue to "splurge" one meal after the next, your recovery from that kind of caloric increase does not come easily. It is much easier to eat calories, than to burn off calories. Consider this fact:

1 pound of fat =3500 calories.

How difficult is it to burn 3500 calories? To walk off one pound of fat (3500 kcal), you would have to walk approximately **14 hours**, at a moderate pace, for approximately **43 miles.** That amounts to a great deal of work AND time! Calories aren't always easy to burn off so be careful when splurging on meals. Thoughtfully choose the foods you eat and snack on during the day when you begin a new exercise regimen. An easy way to ensure success is to have whole foods with every meal. You can decrease your caloric intake while increasing nutrient intake.

- **The Secret**

When you learn how to untie your food and not sabotage yourself just because you ate one "bad" meal, then you will master how to *live* and be healthy all at the same time. For instance, you may have a weekend birthday party to attend around lunchtime. At the party you indulge in a juicy burger along with cake and ice cream for dessert. Absolutely delicious, right? Of course it was! So now what? Do you indulge in calorically high foods for the rest of the day? NO! You can easily recover from this caloric splurge the next time you eat. **Untie your food** by making the next meal cleaner. You found the **secret**! The secret to losing and maintaining your weight over a lifetime is simple: *do not pile one poor meal choice on top of another.* Just do the next right thing. What is the next right thing? A clean, healthy meal that follows. Applying this simple concept is the means to having a healthier body.

Using discipline to untie your food is empowering. It gives you confidence about your health as well as builds confidence within yourself. You know you can splurge on certain foods but effectively get back on track. Expect to indulge in the guilty food pleasures you love every now and then. You do not have to deprive yourself all the time. Choose wisely and respect food and the power that it can have over your health.

Instilling this kind of discipline into your life and making good decisions about the foods you eat will help you feel better. Discipline can be viewed as a faithful friend who will introduce you to your true self. Discipline protects you from an unhealthy life and challenges you to become a better version of yourself and all God created you to be.

Suggestions for not tying your food together

❖ *Pick **one meal** to splurge on, not one **day.***

❖ *Decrease sodium levels after a high sodium meal.*

❖ *Put time and energy into planning your meals.*

❖ *Drink lots of water 1 hour after a splurge meal.*

❖ *You reap what you sow. When you sow good seeds (by making healthier choices) you will reap a harvest of good health.*

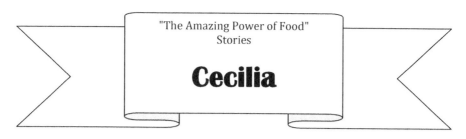

"The Amazing Power of Food"
Stories

Cecilia

"If I can do it, anyone can do it!" says Cecilia, another one of my clients. Cecilia was 59 and had tried many diets in the past. She had never lost more than 15 pounds and always gained back any weight she ever lost. She said, "If this can work for me then it can work for anyone. I promise you I will be your biggest challenge."

Well, three short months later Cecilia was 30 pounds lighter and a year later is holding steady. More noticeable than the pounds that were lost is the confidence she has gained and the freedom she possesses to live a fit and active lifestyle.

*"The simplicity of The Amazing Power of Food menu and the way the information is presented is what makes the difference between this program and other clean eating programs," she says. Cecilia realizes how important eating the right food can be to her overall health and weight. She now has the stamina to exercise on a daily basis, which is something she never did in the past. She cycles, lifts weights, runs, participates in many group exercise classes and is simply UNSTOPPABLE. She never thought a lifestyle change like this was possible or attainable until now. She feels younger and more fit than ever before. Cecilia proves that my favorite saying, once again, remains true: **"I did what I could with what I knew; when I knew better, I did better."***

Chapter 7
You Must Learn More

Now that you have uncovered how to untie your food, and you have thrown away all excuses to eat poorly, it is time you learn more about the food you eat. Knowledge is power. You need to understand how your body reacts to certain foods in order to make better decisions.

- **You Are What You Eat**

    Your body renews its structures daily. Actually, every minute, some renewal is occurring. You are a collection of molecules, cells, tissues, organs, etc., all of which need nutrients. On a cellular level you are exactly what goes into your body. That's right, as cliché as it sounds, *you are what you eat*.

    Every red blood cell in your body regenerates within 120 days. So if your body can only create new cells with the building blocks you feed yourself, you could be building a foundation based on processed garbage.

    The food you eat provides not only energy, but also nutrients. Too little, too much, or simply the wrong foods can all present risks to your health and well-being. If Twinkies and Gummy Worms go into your body, those become the building blocks of your cells. Have you ever seen anything remotely like a Gummy Worm flourishing in nature? But do you think twice about feeding kids gummy products? Now you will. What goes in your mouth today literally becomes the very essence of who you will become tomorrow. Gummy worms, anyone? Luckily, the same principle will help us reshape our health.

- **The Three Letter Word**

I'm sure at one time or another you got that uncomfortable talk about a certain three-letter word. Well, if no one ever sat you down and explained how things work, I guess it's time. Let's talk about **f-a-t**. There are good fats, bad fats, trans fats, saturated fats, monounsaturated fats, and polyunsaturated fats. But for now I want to focus on trans fats. These are not fats that are gender-confused. They are, however, an abomination to all things healthy.

Trans fats (aka trans fatty acids) are a man-made, synthetic fat that is solid at room temperature much like saturated animal fat. Unlike trans fats, saturated animal fat can be found in nature; trans fats are manufactured. To create trans fats, normal, or naturally occurring fats are pumped full of hydrogen to change their chemical makeup. Adding hydrogen gives the fat a sticky, paste-like consistency. Picture a can of shortening. That murky, white paste is trans fat, also known as hydrogenated oil. Now picture you and a spoon attacking the shortening can. No, you can't picture that, right? But the reality is, when we eat processed products like canned icing, processed cheeses, and even peanut butter we are eating this kind of fat.

Here is the big problem with trans fats: they are not water-soluble and we are 85% water. To be exact, 90% of our blood plasma is water, 30% of our bone is water, and 70% of our muscle is water. Thus, our bodies like foods that are water-soluble. However, this type of fat is not. These fats begin to quickly layer in your arteries, creating a barrier around your cells, preventing nutrients from getting into cells. For this reason they have been given the title of the "dangerous fat." They contribute to making HDL (good cholesterol) and LDL (bad cholesterol) ratios worse.

Trans fats are found in many familiar grocery items, such as Pop Tarts, Wheat Thins, Twinkies, and Little Debbie products. They are also found in crackers, cookies, brownies, cereals, breads, and peanut butter, just to name a few. These fats offer packaged food a long shelf life and give items like icing and peanut butter a spreadable consistency.

So why use trans fats? The food industry wants its products to have a long shelf life. The goal is profit, not consumer health-- companies will lose money if food spoils on the shelves. Have you ever seen a spoiled Twinkie? No, of course not—thanks to trans fats.

Furthermore, food manufacturers and restaurants often cook with hydrogenated oils. Why? This fat is cheap and reusable. It is difficult to avoid trans fats completely, but you can certainly limit how much trans fat/hydrogenated oil you consume.

What is the best way to avoid eating trans fats? Take the extra five or ten minutes to prepare your own food. Your health depends upon it--many diseases are linked to excessive intakes of dietary fat and/or excess body fat.

©T h e A m a z i n g P o w e r o f F o o d

The bottom line is that as consumers we cannot rely on fast-food chains, the food-processing industry, or restaurants to give us the nutrients we desperately need as well as the appropriate amount of daily fat and sodium we should consume. Their goal is not to produce healthy consumers, but to make money. Eating out in restaurants, grabbing a quick fast-food sandwich, or eating packaged food products is understandable only every now and then, NOT for every meal. Ask yourself who is in charge of your health? Would you entrust your health to fast-food chains, restaurants, or the food-processing industry? When you are not in control of your food, you are not in control of your physical health.

FOOD FOR THOUGHT: A food company can claim "0 Trans Fats" simply by changing the serving size. The FDA will allow .5 grams per serving and still let the food claim to be trans fat free per serving.

In conclusion, eliminating as much trans fat from your diet as possible will actually give you tremendous long-term health benefits. One simple way to reduce your trans fat intake is to eliminate or eat less pre-packaged edible products. Replace them with healthy, natural whole foods, such as blueberries, spinach, tomatoes, grapes, carrots, oranges—whatever fruit or vegetable you love. Per calorie, these foods strengthen your body and contain the essential vitamins and minerals you need. Plus, choosing to eat whole foods does not require any heavy lifting or even breaking a sweat. Next time you are tempted to eat a Pop Tart or mindlessly snack on heavily processed crackers or chips, think about your poor little cells being smothered in a layer of lard. That visual usually works for me.

- **Fat As A Fuel**

Fats are not our most readily useable fuel source, so it only makes sense that we eliminate as many trans fats from our meals as possible and limit the amount of other fats we consume. When we move and exercise, we burn calories. Carbohydrates are our bodies preferable fuel source in every calorie burned, not fat. So when we have too many fat grams in our food (and by the way, 2 tablespoons of peanut butter has almost 20 grams of fat), we will not easily convert the fat into usable fuel. Instead, the fats will be stored for later use. Start reading labels and analyze how much fat you actually get in one day. You may be surprised.

- **Sweating The Small Stuff**

When most people start a diet or meal plan to lose weight they often concentrate on the small stuff like insignificant condiments or foods that are labeled "fat free" or "light" as a way to cut calories. Instead of sweating a few calories here and there, we need to consider the habitual offenders—eating late at night and drinking alcohol every evening. These things contribute to weight gain and bad health. Try to stay focused on healthy foods to enrich your health. When you make something like a salad, for instance, use as many colorful vegetables as you can. Foods like spinach, broccoli, tomatoes, and carrots are great examples of nutrient rich, colorful vegetables that aid in improving your health. Stop worrying about the little things, like what dressing you may use. Obviously, you cannot dump a bottle of ranch dressing on a small bed of lettuce and have a healthy meal. But you won't eat the salad if it tastes like a compost heap either. If you don't want to make your own dressing (often a simple mix of oil and vinegar or lemon juice), there are plenty of healthy dressings you can choose from. Bottom line: do what it takes to make a salad palatable while keeping it healthy. Take care of the important details like eating a salad made with whole foods and worry less about the *fat free* dressing and *light* cheeses.

FOOD FOR THOUGHT: Sodium is a silent killer. Excessive sodium is linked to hypertension, high blood pressure, heart disease, fluid retention, and kidney stones.

- **Sodium: We don't need much—under 1800mg/day**

Sodium, an often hidden ingredient in food, has a huge impact on our health causing hypertension and high blood pressure. To learn just how much sodium food contains, you must read the labels. Sodium is hidden in many common foods, especially breads, cheeses, and all processed foods. For example, one ounce of most cheeses contains nearly 300 milligrams of sodium. If you are to limit your sodium intake to 1800 mgs/day, and if one ounce of cheese has 300 milligrams of sodium, you can see how challenging staying within this range can be. In addition, many *light* and *fat free* products contain extra sodium, and sugar, to improve the taste that might have been lost due to the removal of fat.

Your cellular makeup is mostly water, and too much sodium dehydrates your body. You do not operate efficiently when you are dehydrated and that is why being mindful and aware of your sodium intake is so important.

- **MSG: We don't need ANY**

Monosodium Glutamate (MSG) is a chemical flavor enhancer that contains large amounts of sodium. MSG has been around for decades. Although the Food and Drug Administration (FDA) has classified MSG as a food ingredient that's "generally recognized as safe," the use of MSG remains controversial. For this reason, when MSG is added to food, the FDA requires that it be listed on the label.

Over the years, the FDA has received many anecdotal reports of adverse reactions to foods containing MSG. These reactions—known as MSG symptom complex—include the following:

- Headache
- Flushing
- Sweating
- Facial pressure or tightness
- Numbness, tingling or burning in face, neck and other areas

- Rapid, fluttering heartbeats (heart palpitations)
- Chest pain
- Nausea
- Weakness

The only way to prevent a reaction is to avoid foods containing MSG. Most of us have heard that Chinese food contains MSG, but did you know **most** boxed food contains MSG? Most lunch meat, flavored chips, crackers with a salty or cheesy coating will contain MSG. Rice cakes can even contain MSG along with many pre-packaged spices and seasonings. Most restaurants use MSG because it enhances the flavor of their food, keeping it consistently tasty.

Remember, MSG is a chemical containing enormous amounts of sodium. At the least, MSG will leave someone with a feeling of not being satiated, wanting more. Far worse, it can produce migraines, headaches, night sweats, and cause severe dehydration. We need to be mindful of the ingredients in the food we eat. Rather than spend time reading long lists of labels on packaged food, spend time preparing your own food!

- **Micronutrients- Fitting them in your day**

A nutrient is *a substance obtained from food that is used in the body to promote growth and maintenance and/or repair.* Essential nutrients are those that the body cannot make in sufficient quantity to meet physiological needs and which must, therefore, be obtained from food. **Micronutrients are the**

vitamins and minerals found in food.

Since our bodies need micronutrients to run efficiently, foods that contain micronutrients are the key to our overall health and wellness. We need to make sure that the fuel we put in our bodies is rich in micronutrients--vitamins and minerals. Where do we find these micronutrients? Again, we turn to real, whole foods, such as spinach, broccoli, apples, strawberries, blueberries, kiwi, mango that are nutrient dense.

So if we know that a double bacon cheese burger from the burger place is not a healthy choice, but a spinach salad, rich in life-sustaining micronutrients is, why don't we make better choices? One reason is minimalism! Minimalism is a modern philosophy that is destroying our health. *'What is the least that I can do and lose weight?' 'What pill can I take to lose weight without having to work too hard?'* Exerting minimum effort and expecting maximum results. That is minimalism and if we learn to recognize it and realize that the results from minimalism are always minimal, we can avoid wasting time trying to find an easy way out. Minimalism nurtures a lazy attitude toward food choices. *'I'm too busy and therefore don't have the time to prepare foods to eat well'* is another common excuse for convenient poor food choices which sabotages good health. No more excuses! You have to give yourself, as well as your loved ones, a fighting chance at beating this obesity epidemic by supplying foods that are rich in nutrients. Make the necessary time to cut up fresh fruit, make some homemade granola (*see recipe*), and have these foods prepared at home or in your car to feed yourself and your family. If anyone is truly hungry, they will eat what is closest to them, whether it's an apple or french fries. PLAN ahead! Pack the healthy alternative and have it with you. Another bonus--just think of the money you will save! It's a win/win situation!

Eating well in the workplace can be easy too. To begin, try bringing healthy lunch and snack alternatives to the office. Most offices are now equipped with small kitchens or, at least refrigerators where you could store your fresh goodies such as salads, fresh fruits, yogurt, and vegetables. It is ideal to eat a clean, micronutrient-dense lunch so that you do not rely solely on dinner to finally get something green or nutritious into your body. Bringing your lunch to work frees up much of your lunch break. Instead of waiting in a long line at the drive thru you can now spend part of that time doing something to energize the rest of your day OR quiet and calm yourself from an overwhelming morning. Exercise does both!

Exercise is a good habit and good habits create good character just as bad habits create bad character. Instead of eating out every day with coworkers or clients, try spending your lunch break moving more. It could be as simple as a walk around the block or a quick trip to your nearest health club. Invite coworkers or clients to exercise with you. Give it a try. It's easier than you think. People love to receive invitations—even to exercise! We practice this principle at our health club: we know that by inviting someone to a group fitness class or to a seminar we host makes people feel special. Invite, Invite, Invite! Boldly invite people to engage in healthy activities with you. You will be surprised at what a positive influence you can be just by asking. You will also be more inclined to exercise if a friend accompanies you.

- **Macro-nutrients: major food categories**

Macronutrients are the big guys-carbohydrates, proteins, fats, water, and fiber—important and manageable! Unfortunately, many diet programs teach sweating the small stuff, and insist on you counting carbohydrates, proteins, or fats. Trying to count macronutrients daily is way too much work--not a life-long practice someone will commit to long term. Few individuals will count "points" forever, nor will they measure and track every morsel of food they eat. It's just too hard. You must keep it simple.

Carbohydrates are your body's most preferred fuel source; it can use carbohydrates 30-50% faster than it can use fat. In fact, carbohydrates are the brain and nervous system's *only* form of fuel. Plus, to metabolize fat, you must have carbohydrates available. But not all carbohydrates are created equal.

Our bodies need "good" carbohydrates that come from whole foods rather than the "bad" carbohydrates found in processed, packaged foods. Examples of good carbohydrates are fresh fruit, vegetables, oats, whole grains, brown rice, and potatoes just to name a few. Examples of bad carbohydrates are processed boxed foods, white bread, crackers, candy, chocolate and the edible products I mentioned earlier. Edible junk! We need good carbohydrates for our body to function properly so consider the source of your calories and carbohydrates because it matters.

Since **protein** composes 50% of our cells, **protein** is an essential part of your meal plan. But too often people are led to believe that they should follow high protein/low carbohydrate diets. WRONG! If your main focus is to feel good and be well, then AVOID these diets! High protein diets food-eliminating diets we discussed earlier. Eliminating a food group (like carbohydrates) does eliminate calories, for sure, but it does not guarantee fat loss or good health. When you rely solely on protein as your fuel source, you end up tired and fatigued, not to mention likely to get an awful headache. In addition, too much protein can create an excess of uric acid in the body causing metabolic diseases like gout. Any excess macronutrient (protein, carbohydrate, or fat) will store as body fat. It is just unused energy.

There is protein in almost everything we eat. Every piece of cake and every cookie contains protein. The point remains that most people are generally not protein deficient; therefore, these diets can put your body in jeopardy. Rather, we become nutrient-deficient by eliminating fruits and vitamin C, as these diets often require.

In the menu portion of this book you will see how each of these **macronutrients** can be balanced throughout every day and every meal.

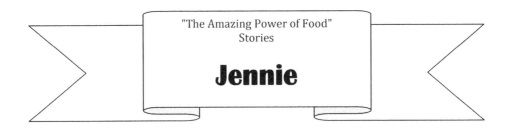

"The Amazing Power of Food"
Stories

Jennie

With three physically demanding jobs, Jennie is always busy and can always use more energy. She works in a chiropractic clinic, has a lawn and garden business, and professionally ropes cattle at rodeo shows throughout Louisiana and Mississippi. Jennie is one of the most inspired, hard-working clients I have ever had the pleasure of working with. I actually met her when I did a nutrition/health seminar at her church. After the seminar she came up to me and told me she wanted to lose a little weight, but more importantly she just wanted to feel better. She was chronically tired and stressed from her workload. So, I introduced her to the Amazing Power of Food program and within a few short weeks she felt remarkably better.

She now has a child-like enthusiasm about eating well and being stronger. Her enthusiasm carries over to her entire family, and she loves sharing all the knowledge she has gained by doing the program. As a result of putting a little effort into preparing meals, Jennie has endless energy from eating well, watching her caffeine and sodium intake, and drinking more water. She knows that preparation is the key to success, so she packs healthy meals and snacks every day to fuel her body the right way. "The time I spend preparing my food is WELL worth the effort" Jennie says. "I wish more people could realize that this one little step (preparation) is the key to being well and strong." Some people have felt bad for so long that they don't know what it feels like to feel good anymore. But by taking the step to prepare your food you can feel better within 24 hours. It's worth a try!

Chapter 8
Steps to Eating Healthier

On a recent afternoon, one of the "regulars" at our health club walked in and greeted me with a flat, monotone "Hi, Julie." Concerned I replied, "How are you doing?" She glumly responded, "Well, I am really tired, and I just don't know why. I have NO energy. I don't even know why I came in today." Since she was a former client of mine I was familiar with how she liked to eat. I asked her "What have you eaten today?" She looked at me sheepishly. "Well, let's see...all I have had is a piece of cornbread and a frappuccino." Not hesitating I said, "Okay, why *should* you feel good? You have had nothing but empty calories--sugar, caffeine, and simple carbohydrates. These foods sap your energy, not replenish it. You have had no REAL nutrition at all." She kind of chuckled and agreed. She knew why she was tired: *How* you eat determines *how* you feel. It still amazes me that people fuel their bodies poorly but still get surprised or concerned when they feel tired and exhausted.

The steps that follow will teach you how to replace your current eating habits with better ones and address most eating challenges. Meal planning tips and guidance will help you make each meal successful. No matter what type of eater you are or what profession you may have, whether you are a full time nurse or a truck driver, you must eat. Don't worry--I am not asking you to become a gourmet chef, expect you to run marathons, or spend tons of money. **However, I do insist that every day you prepare for your success.**

- **STEP 1 – Eat Breakfast**

    Your body, whether or not you think so, wants to be fed in the morning. When you eat breakfast, you inform your body the famine is over; it's time to go to work. When you skip breakfast, your body goes into starvation mode: it reverts to the instincts that have been passed down since the hunt and gather food days. The body thinks it is starved when someone has not eaten for 15 hours (15 hours = eating dinner at 9pm and not eating again until noon the next day). Your body's survival instincts say **"store fat"** so that it can provide energy later. This technique worked effectively when our ancestors could go several days without a meal, a real concern because of food scarcity. However, that is not the case nowadays. How often do you go days without eating food? We know food is very convenient with a fast-food restaurant on almost every corner. When you skip breakfast, you send your body a loud message to store fat, anticipating a starvation event that will never happen.

    A new study from Harvard School of Public Health (HSPH) adds to the evidence that eating breakfast is important for good health. HSPH researchers found that men who regularly skipped breakfast had a 27% higher risk of heart attack or death from coronary heart disease than those who did eat a morning meal. Non-breakfast-eaters were generally hungrier later in the day and ate more food at night, perhaps leading to metabolic changes and heart disease. The study was published July 22, 2013 in the American Heart Association (AHA) journal *Circulation*.

Eating a healthy breakfast is important. It boosts your metabolic rate, helping you burn more calories throughout the day. Eating breakfast basically starts your engine.

Tips for breakfast

1. Plan your breakfast the night before

Before you go to bed, consider what you may eat for breakfast. What you eat for dinner impacts the breakfast you choose. For instance, if you have spaghetti or pizza the night before, a wise choice would be to have egg whites and fresh fruit in the morning. Why? A dinner heavier in carbohydrates needs to be followed up with a high protein, less carbohydrate, less calorie-laden breakfast. On the other hand, if you ate grilled fish, steamed broccoli and a salad for dinner, oatmeal would be a better choice the next morning. Planning the breakfast you will eat ahead of time will help you start your day with the proper nutrients. Breakfast is probably the easiest meal to eat "well" so never miss this opportunity to eat. The 30-Day menu provided in this book is designed to map out these meals for you.

2. Include fresh fruit—it pays high premiums (low-cal/high nutrition)

Unfortunately, most people reach for the same convenient

breakfast every day as they walk out the door. Grabbing a piece of toast, packaged granola bar, or a pop tart for breakfast has become a common choice for many people. A better choice would be to incorporate fresh fruit into every morning meal. Break-the-fast in the morning and choose a well-rounded meal because your body needs vitamins and minerals, not just calories. Your last meal was possibly 9-12 hours earlier and breakfast provides an opportunity to create better health.

Calorie for calorie, fruit delivers maximum nutrition. Most fruits are loaded with the vitamins and minerals we desperately need to be healthy.

Bananas are quite good for you because they have potassium, vitamin C, and other micronutrients. I label bananas the fast-food of fruit because they are easy to eat and peel. However, just like your stock portfolio, you should diversify. Consider the kiwi. A kiwi contains approximately 35 calories, has more vitamin C than an orange, and more potassium than a banana. Such a deal! Eating a variety of fruits will give you the biggest bang for your buck.

3. Preparation is the key

Prepare fresh foods to be readily available. Wash and leave fresh vegetables and fruit in a visible area. You are more likely to eat the foods you see. Invest in a few clear containers and store clean, prepared whole foods in the refrigerator. *Out of sight, out of mind* prevails when foods are hidden. By incorporating fresh fruits every morning with an egg, a couple of egg whites or oatmeal, you have created a powerful breakfast that sets your entire body up for success for the rest of the day.

- **STEP 2- Snack Responsibly--Especially if you are trying to lose weight**

    You should snack a couple times a day if you are feeling a little hungry between meals. You can and sometimes should eat between meals. If you are not hungry two to three hours after your last meal, then you either ate too much at that meal or you haven't moved enough to burn off the calories consumed. Either way, I do not recommend eating a snack shortly after a high calorie breakfast or lunch. Soon you will have a calorie surplus instead of a calorie deficit.

    A snack is just that--a snack. It is not another meal. Keep it relatively small and *less than* **150 calories**. Avoid grabbing empty calories in crackers and pre-packaged low-fat snacks. If you are going to eat, make it count! Please refer to the menus at the back of this book to get healthy snack ideas. Avoid processed carb and fat-laden packaged snack food. If you don't have it in your pantry, you can't mindlessly reach for it—you would have to leave the house to get it and most people will not go to that much effort just for junk food. Think about your goal when you eat a snack. It is to eat well and every choice you make matters. Otherwise, you will revert to the eating habits that lead to an unhealthy body and unhealthy lifestyle.

Be careful while snacking on nuts. Nuts contain fat, and at the end of the day, a fat, is a fat, is a fat. We do not use fat as a readily useable fuel. Even though nuts contain healthy fat, are high in protein and low in carbohydrates, just pay attention to just how many you eat. Many people keep cans of nuts in their desks at work or in their cars to munch on throughout the day. They somehow believe nuts are a "free" snack because they are low in carbohydrates. Because of the high fat content, I recommend that you only have 10-12 nuts in a snack or meal, not several handfuls. The best thing to do is to combine your nuts with an apple or some kind of fresh fruit or vegetable to better satisfy your hunger.

FOOD FOR THOUGHT: A snack is NEVER more than 150 calories.

- **STEP 3 – Lunch**

    Lunch is probably the meal most people look forward to eating, whether it's a meal they eat out, grab along the way, or take time preparing at home. People get excited about the prospects of finally eating a "real" meal. Mid-day eating usually sets the tone for how you will eat for the rest of your day. This is a critical time to make healthy decisions about what and where you will eat.

    Unfortunately, some people choose to skip lunch, thinking they are doing themselves a favor by not eating. They may feel as though they don't have time to eat lunch, or that it is too much of a hassle. I've had clients tell me as soon as they start eating they can't stop, so they choose to not eat , for a while anyway. They plan to have a big dinner to compensate for not having lunch. But skipping lunch will negatively affect your health and your metabolism. First, remember what happens if you skip breakfast; the same thing happens if you skip lunch. If no food is consumed for many hours, the body, starved for nutrition, drops its metabolic rate. Consequences? When you are in starvation mode, you will sabotage good, fundamental decision-making.

Secondly, most people will overeat as soon as they do eat a meal. The body, being loaded with more calories than it can convert to energy, will then store the excess energy(calories) as fat. For your body to be in a state of good health, you want to be able to eat an acceptable amount of calories and use those calories within two to four hours. This is the *healthy* way your body wants to use fuel. When we eat a whopping 1500-2000 calorie meal (many fast-food meal deals are 1500-2000 calories), our bodies cannot efficiently get rid of those calories, not to mention the sodium or the fat found in a meal of that caloric proportion.

If you frequent fast-food restaurants, you can reasonably expect a 1500-2000 caloric-intake in one meal. ONE MEAL = 1500-2000 calories is a fact worth repeating! Yet after consuming ALL THOSE CALORIES how is it possible that you do not feel full or satisfied? You still want some kind of sweet treat or even worse, another meal an hour or so later. How is it possible to feel like there is room for more? The answer is simple. Restaurants often use an enormous amount of fat in the preparation of their food and high fat equals high calories.

- Every gram of fat contains 9 calories.
- Fast-food restaurants use enormous amounts of fat to process their foods.
- Typically, fast-food meal deals have 50-70 grams of fat.
- Do the math: 70 grams of fat multiplied by 9 calories/gram = 630 calories.
- **630 calories from that fast-food meal come straight from fat**.

That number does not include the additional calories found in the remaining carbohydrates and proteins. Relatively small portions of this kind of food can be loaded with calories and fat.

Have you fallen into a sandwich rut at lunchtime? Is lunch not lunch unless it is a sandwich? If your answer is yes, and you are like most people, you will want something crunchy with a sandwich (like a bag of chips) and, of course, wash down that salty goodness with a diet drink or sweetened tea. Well, if this sounds like you, don't be alarmed. You can make sandwiches healthy, but beware of processed lunchmeats and cheeses. Processed lunchmeat always contains extra chemicals, nitrates, coloring, and flavoring to make the flavor and taste consistent. Guess what--even the expensive lunchmeat from the deli is pumped full of the nitrates and preservatives. Think about it. Lunchmeat lasts for months in your refrigerator; just check the "sell by" date. Consider this: If you baked your own chicken or turkey and placed it in your refrigerator, would you eat it 2 weeks later? How about 2 months later? No, I'm sure not. All lunchmeat has a long shelf life due to chemical preservatives. I'm not suggesting that you should never have a sandwich for lunch, but I am suggesting, however, that you should limit your intake of processed meats and cheeses. Fill your sandwiches with fresh vegetables, and if possible, with fresh, not packaged proteins/meats.

Try to pack in as many colorful vegetables as possible at lunch. Tomatoes, broccoli, spinach, shredded carrots, broccoli slaw, cucumbers, and peppers are a few examples of whole foods that contain many antioxidants, vitamins, and minerals that fight disease and taste great with all kinds of salads and even sandwiches. Eat your colorful foods with a lean protein like chicken, turkey, or fish.

PLAN AND PREPARE YOUR LUNCH AHEAD OF TIME. When you plan for a healthy lunch in advance, there will be no questions about the nutritional value, and no worries about eating too much sodium, fat, or calories. Bad decisions lurk around the corner when there is no preparation or little to no thought about what you may eat. Have a plan and practice being prepared.

Tips for lunch:
1. **Eat cleaner proteins**: Lean proteins like chicken, turkey, or fish compliment lunchtime fare like salads and sandwiches. Baking a small turkey breast or roasting a chicken will provide leaner and cleaner proteins throughout the week. These are much better choices compared to processed lunch meats that are full of sodium

and nitrates.

2. Prepare the food: It is always a good idea for busy people to prepare a few meals in advance (usually on the weekends) to make packing your lunch for work a little easier. The menu provided in this book will help take off some of the stress of figuring what you should take to work and help you plan ahead. If your food is prepared all you have to do is grab and go. No thinking, no worrying. Having food pre-made before Monday is just one good decision that will change the rest of your day/week/life! Preparing food is not that time consuming-maybe thirty minutes. That thirty minutes will be spent doing something, so you might as well spend it preparing to be healthier.

- **STEP 4 – Midday Snack**

Watch out—midday snacks can be dangerous territory. Late afternoon could be one of your weakest moments and it's a time that makes sticking to ANYTHING difficult, especially a resolution you made the night before! For most people mid-afternoon is the hardest part of the day to eat well. The hunger sets in, and chips, crackers, and chocolate can tempt you easily at this time of day. *Do not* cave under that pressure. Stay vigilant. Refer to the first snack rule: **A snack is never more than 150 calories; and it must contain real, whole food your body can use as the source of energy you need, now especially** *(Refer to the sample menus in the back of the book for healthy snack ideas).* If you are hungry mid-day, whatever is near will be eaten whether it is french fries or an apple. If you prepare by having that apple or fresh alternative close by a smarter decision can be made.

- **STEP 5- Dinner**

Dinner is the last opportunity for us to eat the vital nutrients we need before we go into our nightly hibernation. It is no mystery that our metabolism slows down at night. When you slow down, your metabolism does as well. Your cells rejuvenate at night, which is another important reason to have good food and nutrients on board.

Portion Control: Since most people overeat at dinner more than any other time during a 24-hour cycle, let's take this opportunity to address the importance of **portion control**. Consuming the right portions ensures proper digestion and elimination of food. Whether you are trying to lose weight or be healthier, your body needs to successfully manage the food you give it 2-4 hours post eating. Below you will find appropriate portion sizes that your body can actually absorb and eliminate in 2-4 hours.

Proteins: When it comes to protein, such as red meat, chicken and fish, the portion size that your body can efficiently digest and use is equivalent to the size of **a deck of cards**. That equates to approximately **4-6 ounces**. That is how much protein you should consume in one meal.

Carbohydrates: The size of your fist is the size of your stomach pouch. A fist-size serving of carbohydrates such as pasta, rice, or potatoes is the perfect portion size for your plate. Again, this is the portion your body can process and efficiently eliminate in 2-4 hours.

You can eat larger portions of whole foods such as freshly steamed broccoli, fresh tomatoes, and spinach because their calories are much lower, and their nutrition per calorie is higher. Indulge: It is perfectly safe to serve yourself larger portions of these foods.

Although you may *want* more than these portion sizes of meat and potatoes, you cannot utilize any more in a 2-4 hour time frame. Staying within these portion guidelines will keep you healthy and as a bonus you will shed any excess fat that your body holds. Closely watching portion sizes will help you lose weight and help prevent diseases such as the all too prevalent Type 2 diabetes. Your body wants to be efficient and work for you. Even though we know moderate portions ensure a healthy body, we often seem to lack the inner strength to make that choice. Adopting this portion-controlled method of eating will nurture you and promote good health.

FOOD FOR THOUGHT: **If your body cannot efficiently eliminate what you ingest, it will store the calories for later use. Watch your portions!**

- **Nighttime snacking**

Dinner is done, the kitchen cleaned, the kids are in bed, and you're ready to collapse on the sofa. It's reward time--time for a snack, right? Wrong! You may feel the need for that edible reward after a long day. Or maybe you just want something to mindlessly munch on because you finally have a moment to yourself. ALERT!! This is not the time to take in more calories. Bedtime is around the corner and your digestive system, along with everything else, just wants to rest. If you fill your body with fuel, your body will be busy digesting food instead of resting.

Have problems sleeping? Did you know that snacks, such as ice cream, wine, or chocolate would cause you to wake up a few hours after falling asleep? The food or beverage you may consume before bedtime can manipulate your blood sugar when you sleep, which interrupts sleep patterns. Sugary snacks like these can also leave you enormously thirsty and dehydrated. I have seen hundreds of people conquer poor sleeping patterns by avoiding late night snacking and drinking. They not only sleep better, they also drop a few pounds in the process!

Timing of dinner does matter: the earlier you can eat dinner, the better. If you have to eat late-eat less. You are about to go to bed anyway so a small amount will do. Becoming a little "empty" before bedtime is ideal. If you eat dinner earlier in the evening, expect to experience small hunger pangs a few hours later. Just think of those pangs as a way of your body talking, telling you "If you don't feed me I will chew off your body fat all night long." It

© T h e A m a z i n g P o w e r o f F o o d

might sound corny, but try it and see. The benefits of going to bed a little empty are enormous. If your body isn't busy digesting and trying to process food, you will sleep better and feel more rested.

Rest is another key component to living a healthy lifestyle and eating less at night will help you rest. Do yourself a favor and don't make it hard on your body at the end of the day by loading up on cups of ice cream, cookies, or alcohol before bedtime. **You have spent all day putting the right fuel in, don't blow it now. Give your body the rest it craves instead of the snacks YOU crave.**

Not only will large dinners and post dinner snacks hinder you from reaching your goal weight, it will keep you from feeling amazing the next day. That extra 300 calorie snack before bedtime equates to someone gaining about 17 pounds a year! Losing weight requires a caloric deficit. You can achieve this deficit by eliminating that after dinner snack only **four** days out of the week. YES—just four or more. The other two or three days out of the week you can freely enjoy a small snack in the evening as long as you keep your snack around 150 calories.

Going to bed at a slight caloric deficit will enable you to wake up and actually *want* a healthy breakfast. Since you did not destructively eat too much the night before, you will look forward to eating. Now you have a brand new opportunity to make healthy food choices. Implementing the steps and guidelines discussed in this chapter will guarantee your success on the healthy path you have chosen.

Roberta

It's 9am and I had just finished teaching a spin class to a dedicated group of Monday morning riders. As I was gathering all of my teaching gear, a woman in my class came up to me and said, "Okay, I have a question for you. Last night I was reading a magazine article that said cycling could make women fat. Is that true?" Before responding, I wondered where she had found that information? But then, as I discuss in the following chapter, I realized how easy it is to become confused because of the deluge of information readily available on the internet, television, or in magazines.

How can people distinguish truth from fiction? I reminded her that you couldn't believe everything you read. I quickly disputed this article and once again explained how you can only gain weight if more calories go in then out. Exercise of any kind cannot make you fat--EVER! It can only help you achieve a calorie deficit that, in turn, can help a person lose weight as long as they don't "eat" their results.

Roberta left class feeling good about her efforts in cycling and even better about understanding what she had read. Be sure to question what you read; don't let confusion stop you from achieving results.

Chapter 9
What to Expect: FAQ's

- **What to expect as you are following the guidelines**

Are you getting pumped to begin this meal plan? I hope so! First, let's examine how you will feel on the first three days of this plan. When you begin eating cleaner food, expect to feel different: Better! More energetic! Amazing!

Day 1 – Start with a healthy breakfast. You incorporate fresh fruit, lean proteins, and healthy complex carbohydrates into your first meal of the day. You then follow this nutritious breakfast with a small, mid-morning snack, a healthy and colorful lunch, eating as many whole foods as possible. A small snack is provided at 3pm in the event you are a little hungry. I guarantee you won't feel that typical mid-afternoon slump you usually feel. A portion-aware dinner follows; be determined to overcome feeling a little empty before bedtime, not starving, just a little empty. Bedtime—What can you expect? **Silent smiles of joy!** You have not succumbed or given into your usual eating patterns. You have kept your promise to yourself. You have ignored the urge to eat. Now how do you feel? Like shouting, "Hooray! I survived DAY 1." Day 1 of the *Amazing Power of Food* is probably more challenging to follow than other days because your body will be adjusting to your new way of eating. Hopefully, your enthusiasm will pull you through. Eat well, go to bed a little empty, and you will wake up feeling a bit deflated, physically, but inflated emotionally. Why deflated physically? Your sodium levels have dropped tremendously, and you will be at a **caloric deficit**. WOW! You will actually *want* to eat breakfast on Day 2. You may not be starving right when you wake up but you will know you need to eat.

FOOD FOR THOUGHT: Nothing will ever *taste* as good as the *feeling* of being healthy and fit.

Day 2- On the second day that you fuel your body properly and apply the principles and meal plan outlined in *The Amazing Power of Food*, you will start to feel different physically because of all the nutrients you have given your body. You will be eager to eat a healthy breakfast and lunch because you ate so well on day one. You should have noticeably more energy on day two. Once again, you eat a portion-aware dinner and go to bed feeling a little empty. Going to bed with a lighter belly brings about positive changes within your body. You will survive these tiny hunger pangs. I have never lost a client due to starvation and I don't anticipate your being the first.

Day 3 – Follow the same schedule as the first two days. When you wake on the third morning of following the *Amazing Power of Food* meal plan, you will feel a difference in your upper mid section. You will not *see* a difference, but you will *feel* the difference. Chances are you will feel less bloated and have even more energy. You have begun to feel better already, and it only took three days of training your body to accept and process the right kinds of food to get you on the right track. You begin to feel the "amazing" part of *The Amazing Power of Food*! Continue to follow the 30-day meal plan day by day. In one short week you will be amazed by how much more energy you have, how little you crave the processed carbohydrate-laden snacks you used to indulge in daily, and how proud you are of the weight you have begun to lose!

Expecting life-changing results is part of being successful in any weight-loss program or change in lifestyle. Sometimes we expect nothing; we just wait to see what happens. Or even worse, we expect to be disappointed because of our past results and behaviors. **Aggressively expect good results**. When you expect to feel better, you will. When you expect the scale to move, it will. You may even exceed your expectations. See yourself in a new way and do not lose sight of that vision. Let's not forget that old saying: "What you see is what you get!"

- **Answering Frequently Asked Questions**

I have been invited to participate in many seminars, panel discussions, corporate office meetings, and/or one-on-one consultations, to answer questions regarding healthy eating. No matter the venue, similar questions about food and exercise arise. I want to share with you the most commonly asked questions and answers.

1. How much water should I drink in a day?

Answer: For general health maintenance, you should consume half of your body weight in ounces of water. So if you weigh 150lbs, you should consume 75 ounces of water daily. Being hydrated or dehydrated greatly affects the way you feel every day. If you exercise, then add an additional 20-24 ounces on that day.

Your exercise intensity and performance are extremely affected by your hydration levels. If you were going on a long road trip, would you fill up your car up with only one fourth of a tank of gas? No! You would prepare your car for the ride and fill the tank to its fullest capacity, wouldn't you? The same principle applies to drinking water. Being fully hydrated when you exercise will lead to improved endurance levels and output.

2. How can I possibly drink that much water?

Answer: Here is a tip; be a destination drinker. For instance, when you know you will be driving somewhere, be that to an appointment or grocery shopping, bring a bottle of water with you and finish the bottle before you get to your destination. Just make sure you are prepared and have the water with you.

Once you have taken in several ounces of water, you do not have to worry about drinking any more for a couple of hours.

FOOD FOR THOUGHT: Drink water. When you think that you have had enough water, drink more water. Water is the essential ingredient to a healthy and fit body. If you feel a little bit thirsty then you are already dehydrated.

3. How bad is caffeine? Can I drink my morning coffee and still lose weight?

Answer: The pros and cons of coffee drinking are vast and confusing, so let's highlight a few facts. First, caffeine will give you a boost of energy, it will slightly raise your metabolism, and it can help your performance athletically. However, too much caffeine *will* raise your blood pressure, suck calcium out of your bones, and leave you dehydrated. So should you drink coffee? Yes, drink it in moderation. For many, drinking a cup of coffee is an essential, not to mention delicious, morning ritual. But think moderation—one or two cups daily will answer your wake up call. Maybe you prefer coffee at lunch? Find the time of the day you need it most, enjoy it, and move on. However, if you have cholesterol or blood pressure issues, staying away from caffeine is a smart and healthy choice for you. Decaffeinated green or herbal teas are a better choice.

Caffeine Content

Type of coffee	Size*	Caffeine**
Espresso, restaurant-style	1 oz. (30 mL)	40-75 mg
Espresso, restaurant-style, decaffeinated	1 oz. (30 mL)	0-15 mg

© T h e A m a z i n g P o w e r o f F o o d

Generic brewed	8 oz. (240 mL)	95-200 mg
Generic brewed, decaffeinated	8 oz. (240 mL)	2-12 mg
Starbucks Latte	16 oz. (480 mL)	150 m
Type of tea	Size*	Caffeine**
Brewed tea		
Black tea	8 oz. (240 mL)	14-61 mg
Black tea, decaffeinated	8 oz. (240 mL)	0-12 mg
Green tea	8 oz. (240 mL)	24-40 mg
Generic instant, unsweetened	8 oz. (240 mL)	26 mg
Lipton Brisk Lemon Iced Tea	8 oz. (240 mL)	5-7 mg
Soft drink	Size*	Caffeine**
Coca-Cola Classic	12 oz. (355 mL)	30-35 mg
Coca-Cola Zero	12 oz. (355 mL)	35 mg
Diet Coke	12 oz. (355 mL)	38-47 mg
Diet Pepsi	12 oz. (355 mL)	27-37 mg
Dr Pepper	12 oz. (355 mL)	36 mg

Mountain Dew	12 oz. (355 mL)	46-55 mg
Pepsi	12 oz. (355 mL)	32-39 mg
Sprite	12 oz. (355 mL)	0 mg

4. "Are diet drinks really bad for you?"

Answer: Unequivocally, YES! Danger, Danger, Danger! Diet drinks consist of phosphoric acid, artificial coloring, and artificial chemical sweeteners dressed up in a refreshing-looking can or bottle. Anyone who has given up diet sodas and regular sodas will testify to feeling 100% better immediately. Artificial sweeteners have been proven to be very dangerous for your overall health. Recent studies show that they can actually increase your appetite.

Artificial sweeteners are chemicals or natural compounds that replace the sweetness of sugar. You have given your vital organs extra work: they *must* filter these chemicals. Just because the FDA approves these artificial sweeteners does not mean you should use them!

The 5, FDA-approved, artificial sweeteners to avoid are as follows:

1- Acesulfame potassium (Sunett)
2- Aspartame (NutraSweet or Equal)
3- Sucralose (Splenda)
4 -D-Tagatose (Sugaree)
5. Saccharin (Sweet 'N Low)

You may be surprised to see saccharin on that list. Discovered in 1879, saccharin, which is 300 times sweeter than sugar, was used during World War I and World War II to make up for sugar shortages and rationing. In the 1970s, the FDA was going to ban saccharin based on the reports of a Canadian study that showed that saccharin was causing bladder cancer in rats. A public outcry kept saccharin on the shelves (there were no other sugar substitutes at that time), but with a warning label that read, "Use of this product may be hazardous to your health. This product contains saccharin which has been determined to cause cancer in laboratory animals." Like saccharin, aspartame is another sweetener that, though thoroughly tested by the FDA and deemed safe for the general population, has had its share of critics who blame the sweetener for causing everything from brain tumors to chronic fatigue syndrome.

Sucralose (otherwise known as Splenda) is even scarier. Recent research suggests that Splenda can enlarge both the liver and kidneys and shrink the thymus glands. Sucralose breaks down into small amounts of dichlorofructose, which has not been adequately tested in humans. Reportedly, Splenda can cause skin rashes, panic, diarrhea, headaches, bladder issues, and stomach pain, just to name a few!

Staying away from eating or drinking artificial sweeteners is always in your best interest. If you do have a diet soda, you should immediately drink just as many ounces of water as you did soda.

For example, if you have a 24 ounce bottle of diet coke, drink 24 ounces of water immediately after. It will help flush some of the chemicals and phosphoric acid out of your body.

Diet soda is 100 percent nutrition-free. Drink water instead! It is just as important to drink water, the good stuff, as it is to avoid the bad stuff. If you take in many ounces of alternative beverages or liquids, you are also limiting your intake of water you would have otherwise drunk. Regular sodas that contain real sugar are just as bad for you, but in a slightly different way. When you drink a regular soda, you consume useless calories (about 270-400 calories, depending on the size of the drink). Sodas do not contain anything nutritionally sound--just simply a waste of calories. If you decide to stop drinking carbonated soda and replace those drinks with water, you will see pound after pound fall off just from eliminating those empty calories.

Food For thought: Diet soda is 100 percent nutrition-free. It is just as important to actively drink water, the good stuff, as it is to avoid the bad stuff. If you are taking in 5-6 cans of soda a day you are also limiting your intake of water you would have otherwise drunk.

5. "I've heard that it is good to drink red wine to lower your cholesterol and get antioxidants. Is this true?"

Answer: Drinking red wine because of its antioxidants has been termed as the "French Paradox." You actually get just as many antioxidants drinking grape juice or eating grapes, but without the metabolic-slowing alcohol. Alcohol is alcohol whether it is found in beer, wine, or liquor.

If you look at alcohol from a calorie perspective, one gram of alcohol has 7 calories: Look at the difference: One gram of a carbohydrate has 4 calories, one gram of protein has 4 calories, and one gram of fat has 9 calories. So you can see how calorically dense alcohol is--almost *double the calories of a carbohydrate or protein*. So those of you who enjoy a glass of wine or two everyday with dinner, please take note. How much wine are you actually drinking? Four ounces? Probably not. Wine glasses these days hold no less than a whopping 8-12 ounces which can pack a big caloric punch to any meal.

Carbohydrates, proteins, and fats can be stored in our bodies, but alcohol cannot. For this reason it takes priority over everything else until it is metabolized. The consequences? All other processes that are supposed to be happening in your body are suppressed. They take a backseat until the alcohol has been metabolized. Plus, alcohol acts strangely in your system. Your body will choose to oxidize alcohol instead of fat. "Alcohol spares fat" according to studies. Therefore, ingesting alcohol is similar to consuming quantities of dietary fat.

If that still doesn't help you think twice about your alcohol consumption, this might. Alcohol destroys the vitamin B complex group, vitamins A and C, as well as zinc, magnesium, and calcium. It stimulates the kidneys to excrete more fluid than you take in, which can create a relative state of dehydration—especially dangerous for someone who sweats quite a bit on a regular basis. To sum it up, alcohol should be consumed only in extreme moderation. If being healthy and losing weight are your goals, drinking alcohol everyday will NEVER allow you to reach them.

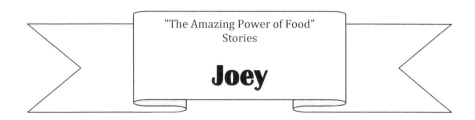

"The Amazing Power of Food"
Stories

Joey

Joey, 23, has lost 107 lbs in one short year, and he has created a new life for himself. From the time he was a child, he has always battled his weight. Fed up and ready to change, Joey decided to start the Amazing Power of Food program under the recommendation of his sister. She had less weight to lose than Joey, but achieved her personal goal, losing more than 20 pounds. She did the program three years before and has successfully kept the weight off. How did Joey lose over 100 pounds without surgery? By following the same guidelines provided in this book. What did Joey do to keep him going? How did he create such a powerful environment for success? He attributes his success to two things: 1) being patient for results and 2) doing away with all of the excuses he used in the past. "I learned that dieting doesn't mean you can't eat," Joey says. "The Amazing Power of Food menus were easy to follow. There is not a lot of prep time or cooking involved either. I love whole foods now and look forward to every meal I eat. I can fix a full plate of food and still maintain a calorie deficit."

Joey did what I asked him to do-**trust the process!** He wasn't a slave to the scale and knew that weighing himself every day would only discourage and/or encourage him the wrong way. Let me *explain; we do not pick and chose when fat (or weight) comes off or on. Our bodies are funny that way. You can work hard for weeks and "weigh-in" every day only to be disappointed because your weight hasn't budged. That is **dis**couraging. But one day you step on the scale and BAM-you lost 4-6 pounds! Results can show up overnight, but they weren't achieved overnight for sure. On the flip side, you can eat poorly for days, "weigh-in" every day and to your surprise, the scale hasn't budged. You're excited! That's **en**couraging, right? Sure it is. Then one day as you habitually weigh-in, you gasp at your 8-pound weight gain. The scale encouraged you when it shouldn't have. It happens all the time. Don't be a slave to the scale. Follow the menu and trust the process!*

Chapter 10
The Weight Loss Equation

Watching people becoming healthier over the last thirty years has surely been rewarding for me, and the science and secrets behind their success are pretty simple. Forget the myriad of special diet books, gimmicks, and counting whatever plans--life is complicated enough. Losing weight is simple; we just have to do the basic math. Math? Already, I feel you squirming. I know, math is a four-letter word in my house, too. But here is the basic equation:

3500 calories = 1 lb. If you want to lose one pound of fat, no matter how old you are, you have to be at a caloric deficit of 3500 calories. Many people think that once they turn forty or fifty years old, their metabolism takes a u-turn and slows down right then and there. Not true. As you age *you* may slow down, which can slow your metabolic rate, but your metabolism does not have a dimmer switch that goes down as soon as you turn fifty. So ladies, if turning fifty or going through menopause has been your reason for gaining ten or more pounds, you need to find a more valid excuse. Age has nothing to do with it at all. Whether you are 8 years old or 80 years old, **you must be at a caloric deficit to lose weight--period!**

If you are wanting to lose a pound a week, and you normally take in an average of 2000 calorie per day, by simply cutting out one large soft drink (approximately 250 calories) and going for a thirty minute walk (burning approximately 250 calories), you have eliminated 500 calories in one day! Your caloric intake went from 2000 calories to 1500 calories. Watch this math: That simple exchange equals a 3500-calorie deficit over one week. **Remember**: 3500 calories = one pound of fat. In approximately one week, you will lose one pound. If we multiply those figures, in one year you can lose over 20 pounds, if not more, that easily. Beware, the opposite of this can happen just as easily. If you take **in** 3500 calories more than you burn per week, you will gain a pound of fat. It is that simple. So it is up to you how quickly you gain or lose weight. Keeping in mind that calories do matter, you want a majority of your calories to come from super foods--real, whole foods that provide your body with the nutrients it needs to function at peak performance. Plan on plenty of complex carbohydrates and good lean proteins. You will then be taking in fewer calories, but more nutrients.

The bottom line to losing weight is finding *your* way to be at a caloric deficit. This book offers the guidelines to make that caloric deficit a healthy one.

Living your life in good health does not happen by accident. You must plan and prepare to be healthy. Ask anyone who is in good health. They all practice healthy habits, and quite frankly, they love to share their secrets. I enjoy asking elderly people who are in good health what their secrets are, and it always comes down to three things. They stay physically active (keep moving), eat well a majority of the time (usually eating smaller portions), and remain somewhat social. These three things create an

© T h e   A m a z i n g   P o w e r   o f   F o o d

environment for physical success. People who remain in good health pursue good health. It is never too late and never too difficult. You can feel 30 at the age of 75, but to get there every meal counts. The amazing power of the food you eat will be the building blocks for your new, healthy life.

Everyone can achieve weight loss and good health. I don't know how else to say it. If you want to lose weight and be in good health, and if you can manage to maintain a little self-discipline, you **will** succeed. I know it. I have seen it. *The Amazing Power of Food* is more than a book with some menus and facts. *The Amazing Power of Food* gives you a common sense approach to good health and wellness. The menus provided are simple and easy to follow. Complicated recipes and food choices would simply discourage you. This 30-day menu is an easy and effective plan for losing weight and becoming healthier.

To help you get started, I have also included a grocery list. You don't have to shop at specialty stores; these foods are common foods you can get at your local supermarket. Following this menu to a "t" (eating meals in the order provided) will help you achieve real results relatively fast. This menu is not wasteful. You may see repeat items within a few days so that you do not waste any food or money. In addition, you will find easy-to-follow recipes and a daily log sheet if you want to log the food you eat. Planning does not get easier than this. It's time to put on your shoes, go to the store, and get ready to feel completely rejuvenated!

Weekly Grocery List

Produce:

Fresh spinach
Mixed greens
Tomatoes
Red bell pepper
Green bell pepper
Yellow bell pepper
Orange bell pepper
Red onion
White onion
Celery
Jalapeño pepper
Broccoli Slaw
Carrots (shredded, baby, or whole)
Mushrooms
Potatoes
Broccoli
Avocado
Cucumber
Kiwi
Apples
Blueberries
Blackberries
Strawberries
Bananas
Lemons
Limes
Seasonal fruit
Garlic

Protein:

Chicken breast
Ground turkey breast or whole turkey
Lean ground beef
Tuna filet
Salmon filet
Mahi Mahi (or white flaky fish)
Eggs

Other Foods:

Low calorie bread
Pizza Crust
Pasta
Brown rice
Black beans
Edemame (soybeans)
Rotel (canned diced tomatoes)
Spaghetti sauce
Nuts
Oatmeal
Maple syrup
Molasses
Peanut Butter -Natural
Cream Cheese (low fat)
Sour cream - Light
Greek yogurt
Skim milk
Green decaffeinated tea
Cinnamon
Pizza sauce

The amount of food you purchase depends on the number of people you need to feed. The more people, the more produce. Give or take a few items, this grocery list will help you create delicious meals every week. The foods listed above will help you make many of the recipes found in this book.

The Amazing Power of Food©

30-Day Meal Plan

Day 1

Breakfast	1 egg 2 egg whites scrambled or hard boiled 1 cup of fresh fruit (1/2 small apple, strawberries and kiwi)
Snack	10 almonds 1 small apple
Lunch	Large Mixed Green Salad (see recipe)
Snack	Brown rice cake with 1 tbsp almond butter
Dinner	4-6 oz. grilled or baked chicken breast 1 cup (or more) lightly steamed broccoli Fresh tomatoes drizzled with vinegar, 1tsp. extra virgin olive oil ½ cup pasta prepared any way

*Prepare to feel a little hungry at certain times on this day. You should be at a caloric deficit and typically sodium levels are much lower than normal. Drink lots of water.

Day 2

Breakfast	Oatmeal (use real oatmeal, not instant – 1 serving as shown in directions) 1 banana
Snack	½ cup strawberries ½ cup Greek yogurt
Lunch	4-6 oz. grilled tuna filet Small mixed green salad 1 orange

Snack	1 apple
	1 tsp. peanut butter
Dinner	Pasta salad (see recipe)

Day 3

Breakfast	4 oz. yogurt (brand of your choice)
	½ cup blueberries, ½ cup strawberries
	¼ cup of granola (see recipe)
Snack	2 hard-boiled eggs – 1 yolk only
Lunch	Turkey and veggie wrap (see recipe)
	1 orange or apple
Snack	No snack
Dinner	Black beans and brown rice (see recipe)
	Small Mixed Green Salad

Day 4

Breakfast	1 egg and 2 whites scrambled or hard-boiled
	1 cup of fresh fruit (ex...mango, kiwi, oranges and apples)
Snack	1 apple with 10 nuts of your choice
Lunch	Pasta salad (see recipe)
Snack	1 banana
Dinner	4-6 oz. baked or grilled fish of your choice
	Wilted spinach (see recipe)
	Sautéed squash and zucchini
	½ cup brown rice

Day 5

Breakfast	*½ whole wheat bagel with 1 tbsp. cream cheese* *½ cup fresh strawberries*
Snack	*1 apple*
Lunch	*Fresh spinach salad with 4-6 oz. grilled chicken (see recipe)*
Snack	*2 hard boiled eggs (1 yolk)*
Dinner	*4-6 oz. filet mignon* *1 cup fresh steamed broccoli – season to taste* *1 fresh tomato sliced* *Baked potato (size of your fist) – dressed with green onions, 1 oz. cheese, 1 tsp. sour cream*

Day 6

Breakfast	*Power Smoothie (see recipe)*
Snack	*1 hardboiled egg*
Lunch	*Tuna or chicken salad in a pita pocket (see recipe)*
Snack	*1 apple*
Dinner	*Black or red beans with brown rice* *Lightly steamed asparagus with lemon juice*

Day 7

Breakfast	Oatmeal (use real oatmeal, not instant – 1 serving as shown in directions) ¼ cup blueberries ½ sliced apple
Snack	No snack
Lunch	Turkey Veggie Sandwich (see recipe for Turkey veggie wrap and replace with low-cal bread)
Snack	2 raw carrots (peeled and chopped into sticks) 2 tbsp. hummus
Dinner	Chicken spaghetti (see recipe) 1 cup spaghetti squash (see recipe) Small green salad

Day 8

Breakfast	1 cup Granola (see recipe) ½ cup skim milk (pour over granola) ½ cup fresh berries
Snack	1 hardboiled egg
Lunch	Power Smoothie (see recipe)
Snack	Brown rice cake 1 tbsp almond butter
Dinner	4-6 oz. grilled tuna or salmon filet Large Mixed Green Salad 1 whole grain roll

Day 9

Breakfast	*1 egg with 3 egg whites scrambled or hard-boiled* *1 mango or 1 whole grapefruit*
Snack	*½ cup granola*
Lunch	*Turkey Veggie Sandwich (see recipe)* *2 carrots (peeled and chopped into sticks)*
Snack	*1 apple* *10 nuts*
Dinner	*Chicken Stir fry (see recipe)* *1 cup brown rice*

Day 10

Breakfast	*Oatmeal (use real oatmeal, not instant – 1 serving as shown in directions)*
Snack	*No snack*
Lunch	*Pasta Salad (see recipe)*
Snack	*1 apple, 1 banana*
Dinner	*Veggie pizza (see recipe)-2 slices* *Small green salad*

Day 11

Breakfast	*4oz. yogurt (preferably Greek yogurt)* *½ cup strawberries* *½ cup blueberries and blackberries*
Snack	*No snack*
Lunch	*Chicken Vegetable Sandwich (see recipe for Chicken/Turkey Vegetable Sandwich)*
Snack	*1 apple* *10-12 Nuts*
Dinner	*Spaghetti – Make your favorite red sauce (can include chicken or meat) and serve over 1 cup cooked pasta* *Fresh broccoli- lightly steamed*

Day 12

Breakfast	*1 egg 2 whites scrambled* *1 banana*
Snack	*1 mango* *10 nuts*
Lunch	*2 pieces of Veggie pizza*
Snack	*½ cup granola* *1 apple*
Dinner	*Ground turkey breast burger (see recipe)* *Steamed or roasted veggies (see recipe)*

Day 13

Breakfast	*1 piece toast (or 1/2 bagel) with 1 tsp. peanut butter* *1 grapefruit*
Snack	*No snack*
Lunch	*Tuna salad (see recipe) – serve on a fresh spinach salad* *5 multi grain crackers*
Snack	*4 oz. yogurt (preferably Greek yogurt)* *1 apple*
Dinner	*Black beans and Brown rice (see recipe)* *Cucumber, celery, onion salad (see recipe)*

Day 14

Breakfast	*Oatmeal (use real oatmeal, not instant – 1 serving as shown in directions)*
Snack	*No snack*
Lunch	*Turkey vegetable sandwich* *1 orange*
Snack	*2 hard-boiled eggs (1 yolk)* *10 carrot sticks* *2 tbsp. hummus*
Dinner	*Power Smoothie (see recipe)*

Day 15

Breakfast	1 egg 2 whites scrambled ½ cup strawberries ½ cup blueberries
Snack	1 green apple ¼ cup granola
Lunch	Tuna salad (see recipe) or 4oz. tuna filet on Spinach Salad (see recipe)
Snack	No snack
Dinner	4-6 oz. chicken breast 1 cup of fresh lightly steamed broccoli 4 slices tomato with 1oz. feta cheese (sprinkle feta on top and drizzle with balsamic vinegar) 1/2 cup of pasta- prepared any way

Day 16

Breakfast	Whole-wheat toast with peanut butter 1 tbsp. cottage cheese 1 tbsp. fig (or your favorite) preserves-layer all ingredients on toast
Snack	1 banana ½ cup granola (see recipe)
Lunch	Chicken salad (see recipe)
Snack	1 green apple
Dinner	4-6 oz. grilled fish Steamed asparagus Small green salad

Day 17

Breakfast	*Egg McMuffin (see recipe)*
Snack	*1 orange*
Lunch	*Soybeans with stir fry (see recipe)*
Snack	*1 cup of yogurt* *½ cup blueberries*
Dinner	*4-6 oz. Grilled fish* *Fresh steamed broccoli* *Fresh tomatoes with 1 oz. mozzarella cheese* *½ cup brown rice*

Day 18

Breakfast	*2 whole-wheat Kashi waffles*
Snack	*1 grapefruit* *10-12 nuts*
Lunch	*Veggie pizza–2 pieces (see recipe)* *Small green salad*
Snack	*1 kiwi* *½ cup granola*
Dinner	*Spaghetti (1 cup of pasta) with your favorite spaghetti sauce* *Steamed broccoli*

Day 19

Breakfast	*Fresh fruit* *1 egg with 2 whites omelet*
Snack	*1 nectarine, 1 kiwi* *10-15 Almonds*
Lunch	*Tuna filet* *Spinach salad*
Snack	*No Snack*
Dinner	*2 Grilled Chicken Soft Tacos (see recipe)*

Day 20

Breakfast	*Power Smoothie (see recipe)*
Snack	*1 large apple*
Lunch	*Turkey Veggie Sandwich in a pita pocket (or light whole wheat bread)* *1 orange*
Snack	*1cup Greek yogurt* *½ cup strawberries or 1 banana*
Dinner	*Salmon Filet* *Spinach salad (see recipe)*

© T h e   A m a z i n g   P o w e r   o f   F o o d

Day 21

Breakfast	*Oatmeal (use real oatmeal, not instant – 1 serving as shown in directions)* *¼ cup blueberries*
Snack	*No snack*
Lunch	*2 grilled chicken soft tacos*
Snack	*1 apple*
Dinner	*4-6 oz. filet mignon* *1 cup fresh steamed broccoli – season to taste* *1 fresh tomato sliced* *Baked potato (size of your fist) – dressed with green onions, 1 oz. cheese, 1 tsp. sour cream*

Day 22

Breakfast	*1 Breakfast Egg Burrito (see recipe)*
Snack	*No snack*
Lunch	*Power Smoothie*
Snack	*1 apple* *1 tsp. peanut butter*
Dinner	*Vegetable Soup (see recipe)*

Day 23

Breakfast	Whole-wheat toast with peanut butter 1 tbsp. cottage cheese 1 tbsp. fig preserves-layer all ingredients on toast
Snack	1 orange
Lunch	Vegetable soup 5 whole grain crackers
Snack	½ cup granola
Dinner	Black beans and Brown rice (see recipe) Cucumber, celery, onion salad (see recipe)

Day 24

Breakfast	Egg McMuffin (see recipe)
Snack	No snack
Lunch	4-6 oz. chicken breast 10 carrot sticks-2 tbs. hummus 1 tomato sliced ½ avocado ½ cup black bean salsa (see recipe)
Snack	1 apple
Dinner	Vegetable soup- 1 large bowl 1 whole grain roll

Day 25

Breakfast	*4 oz. yogurt (preferably Greek yogurt)* *½ cup strawberries* *½ cup blueberries and blackberries*
Snack	*½ bagel* *1 tsp. cream cheese*
Lunch	*Chicken salad (see recipe) on bed of fresh spinach*
Snack	*No snack*
Dinner	*4-6 oz. grilled mahi mahi (or another white flaky fish)* *1 cup black bean salsa* *½ avocado* *Fresh tomatoes*

Day 26

Breakfast	*Oatmeal - (use real oatmeal, not instant – 1 serving as shown on directions)* *¼ cup berries*
Snack	*½ cup non-fat Greek yogurt* *Fresh berries*
Lunch	*PB&J sandwich on whole wheat* *1 apple*
Snack	*No snack*
Dinner	*4-6 oz. Grilled Chicken breast* *Spinach salad (see recipe)*

Day 27

Breakfast	Whole-wheat toast with 1 tsp peanut butter
	1 tbsp. cottage cheese
	1 tbsp. fig preserves-layer all ingredients on toast
	1 kiwi
Snack	No snack
Lunch	Power Smoothie
Snack	½ cup granola
Dinner	4-6 oz. grilled fish
	Steamed asparagus or broccoli
	Small green salad

Day 28

Breakfast	Fresh fruit
	1 egg with 2 whites omelet
Snack	10-12 nuts of your choice
	1 handful pretzels
Lunch	Mixed green salad (see recipe)
Snack	No snack
Dinner	Pasta Salad (see recipe)

Day 29

Breakfast	1 cup granola 1 apple
Snack	No snack
Lunch	4-6 oz. chicken breast 10 carrot sticks-2 tbs. hummus 1 tomato sliced ½ avocado ½ cup black bean salsa (see recipe)
Snack	No snack
Dinner	Ground turkey breast burger (see recipe) Steamed or roasted veggies (see recipe)

Day 30

Breakfast	4oz. yogurt (preferably Greek yogurt) 1 grapefruit
Snack	1 apple 1 tbsp. peanut butter
Lunch	Tuna salad on bed of mixed greens
Snack	1 cup mixed fruit 10 Walnuts or almonds
Dinner	Mixed green salad (see recipe)

ALMOND CRANBERRY GRANOLA
4 cups oatmeal
1 cup almonds (or nut of choice)
¼ cup molasses, ¼ cup maple syrup, 1 tbsp. honey
1 tbsp. cinnamon
¼ teaspoon vanilla extract
¼ tsp. salt
dried fruit (optional)
Heat molasses, maple syrup, honey vanilla extract and add salt.
Combine oats, nuts, cinnamon, and heated mixture until
ingredients are thoroughly combined. Spread on a cookie sheet
and bake at 375 for 10 minutes stir and bake another 5-7 minutes.
Completely cool and store in airtight container.

BLACK BEANS AND BROWN RICE
1 can of black beans (drained)
1 can Rotel Tomatoes (drained)
¼ onion (chopped)
½ fresh tomato (chopped)
1 tbsp. sour cream
Brown Rice
Drain and rinse 1-8 oz. can of black beans. Heat in a small
saucepan. Add 1 can of diced Rotel Tomatoes to beans. Serve 1 cup
of beans and 1 cup of brown rice. Top with 1 tbsp. sour cream,
onions and fresh tomatoes. Makes 2-3 servings.

BLACK BEAN SALSA

2 cans black beans (drained and rinsed)
1 bell pepper, chopped
6 roma tomatoes, chopped
1 red onion, chopped
1-4 oz. corn
2 limes (freshly squeezed)
3 tbsp. balsamic vinegar
1 tsp. olive oil
Salt and pepper to taste

BREAKFAST EGG BURRITO

3 egg whites
Onions
Fresh spinach
Fresh tomatoes
Mushrooms
Garlic, chopped
1oz. cheddar cheese
1 flour tortilla or corn tortilla
1 tbsp. salsa
Salt and pepper to taste
Lightly spray a skillet with non- stick cooking spray. Sauté all vegetables then add egg whites. Cook thoroughly and place in flour or corn tortilla. Sprinkle with cheese and salsa, roll up and enjoy!

CHICKEN SALAD
4-6 oz. chicken (shredded)
¼ cup celery (finely chopped)
¼ cup carrots (finely chopped)
1 tbsp. Greek Yogurt
1 tsp. mayo
½ tbsp. mustard
Sliced grapes (optional)
Season to taste
Mix all ingredients and season to taste. Serve over a bed of mixed greens of in a pita pocket

CHICKEN SPAGHETTI
(2) 4 -6 oz. chicken breast chopped
1 tbsp. olive oil
½ onion
4 cloves garlic
1 can diced tomatoes
1 jar of spaghetti sauce

Sauté onions and garlic in olive oil and add chicken. Combine diced tomatoes and sauce and serve over pasta or squash. Makes 3-4 servings.

CHICKEN STIR-FRY
4- 6 oz. Chicken
1/2 onion
3 cloves garlic
1 green and red pepper
2 carrots sliced
½ cup mushrooms
3 stalks broccoli
1 cup edamame
3 tbsp. Soy sauce
1 tsp. sesame oil
3 tbsp. rice wine vinegar

Salt and pepper to taste
Sauté onions, garlic and peppers with sesame
oil in skillet. Add chicken and other seasonings
(soy sauce, rice wine vinegar). Cook over medium
heat 6-7 minutes or until thoroughly cooked.
Remove chicken and add remaining vegetables.
Lightly cook vegetables and add chicken back
in skillet. Cook for 2 minutes and serve over 1/2 cup rice.
Makes 3-4 servings.

CHICKEN/TURKEY VEGETABLE SANDWICH

1- 4 oz. chicken breast or roasted turkey breast
1 handful mixed greens
1oz. cheese
1/2 sliced tomato
1/4 thinly sliced red bell pepper
1/4 thinly sliced avocado
2 slices whole wheat bread
Dress with mustard or ketchup (optional)

CUCUMBER CELERY ONION SALAD

Chop all three ingredients and drizzle 1 tsp. olive oil and vinegar.
Salt and pepper to taste.

EGG MCMUFFIN

1 whole wheat English muffin
1 egg
1oz. cheese
1slice of ham
Cook 1 egg and place on toasted English muffin.
Top with cheese and ham while warm.

EGG WHITE OMELET

1 egg, 2egg whites
2 tbsp. milk
2 handfuls spinach
Fresh tomatoes (chopped)
3 mushrooms(chopped)
1 handful broccoli slaw
Sprinkle of parmesan cheese

GRILLED CHICKEN SOFT TACOS

4-6oz. chicken breast
¼ cup chicken broth
2 flour or corn tortillas
Red bell pepper, sliced
Yellow bell pepper, sliced
Onions, sliced
Carrots, sliced
Avocado, sliced
1 tsp. sour cream
1 oz. cheddar cheese
Fresh spinach (chopped)
Fresh tomatoes
1 tsp. chili powder or taco seasoning
¼ tsp. garlic powder
Salt and pepper to taste

Sauté peppers, onions, and carrots in chicken stock. Season vegetables. Remove vegetables and set aside. Add chicken and seasoning. Simmer until thoroughly cooked. Add vegetables back to skillet and sauté for 2 minutes. Dress each taco with chicken, vegetables, fresh spinach, tomatoes, sour cream, and cheese.

MIXED GREEN SALAD

2 handfuls spinach
1 handful mixed greens
Vegetables – carrots, cucumber, tomato, avocado, red bell pepper...
1oz. cheese
¼ cup edamame (soy beans), garbanzo beans, or black beans
Lemon juice
1 tbsp. dressing of your choice
Mix all ingredients together and squeeze lemon juice over salad
then add dressing of your choice

PASTA SALAD

1 cup whole grain/wheat pasta
4-6 oz. cooked chicken breast, diced
Diced carrots
Diced broccoli
Fresh spinach leaves
Red onion chopped
Red pepper chopped
1 tbsp. lemon juice
1 tbsp. italian dressing
Parmesan cheese

POWER SMOOTHIE

¼ cup skim milk
¼ cup Greek yogurt
¼ cup oats
¼ cup strawberries
¼ cup blueberries
½ banana
1 tsp. peanut butter
1 tsp. honey
Ice
Blend all ingredients with ice and serve.

ROASTED VEGETABLES

Fresh vegetables- broccoli, onions,
mushrooms, asparagus bell pepper (red, orange, yellow),
zucchini, squash and any other veggie of choice.

2 tbsp. olive oil
2 tbsp. vinegar
¼ tsp lemon pepper
1/8 tsp. sea salt
Pepper

Place cut vegetables in large bowl. Add olive oil and seasonings
and toss vegetables.
Layer vegetables on baking sheet and roast in oven 10-12 minutes.

SALAD DRESSING:

¼ cup olive oil
½ cup red wine vinegar
¼ cup balsamic
4 cloves of garlic, finely chopped
3 tsp. dijon mustard
1 tsp. salt
6 dashes Worcestershire sauce
Juice of 1 lemon

SPAGHETTI SQUASH

1 spaghetti squash
1 tbsp. olive oil
Salt and pepper to taste

Cut squash in half and take out seeds. Place squash face
down on cookie sheet and bake at 400 degrees for 20-25 min.
Remove squash from oven. Using a fork, slide fork through
squash and squash will resemble spaghetti noodles.
Lightly season squash with olive oil, salt, and pepper.
Serve in place of pasta.

EDAMAME (SOYBEANS) WITH STIR-FRY
Same as chicken stir-fry just replace chicken with 2 cups soybeans

SPINACH SALAD
2 large handfuls of fresh spinach
Carrots
Tomatoes
Mushrooms
Cucumbers
Red onion
Red or green grapes
1oz. Feta (or favorite) cheese
Place chicken on 2 large handfuls
of spinach, all veggies chopped and sprinkle
with 1oz. of your favorite cheese.

TURKEY BREAST BURGER
4-6 oz. ground turkey breast
Lettuce
Onion
Tomato
Fresh greens
Season to taste.
Make patties and sauté in skillet until thoroughly cooked.
Serve on a whole-wheat bun-dress with lettuce,
onion, tomato, fresh spinach or greens, mustard, and ketchup.

TURKEY VEGGIE WRAP
4 oz. shredded turkey meat
Small handful of spinach
Small handful of broccoli slaw
Shredded carrots
Fresh tomatoes
Red onion
1 oz. cheese (your favorite)
1 spinach wrap or lavish wrap
1 tsp. honey mustard or low fat ranch dressing
Dress the wrap with your favorite veggies and turkey
Roll up and enjoy!! Makes 2 servings

TUNA SALAD
8 oz. tuna
2 boiled egg whites
¼ cup Greek yogurt
1 tbsp. mayo
¼ onion, chopped
2 stalks celery, chopped
¼ cup chopped carrots or apples (optional)
2 tbsp. dill relish
Season to taste
(Makes 3-4 servings)

VEGETABLE SOUP
1 large onion
4 stalks celery
6 roma tomatoes
1 zucchini
1 cup cabbage
Broccoli
3 cups fresh spinach
2 cups frozen edamame

5 cloves garlic
4 oz. corn (optional)
8 oz. chicken or vegetable broth
1 tsp. cayenne pepper
Salt and pepper to taste
Water

Combine all ingredients in pot. Add broth, water (as much water as broth) and seasonings. Simmer and serve!

VEGGIE PIZZA

1 Mama Mary's Pizza Crust(or thin crust of any kind)
½ jar Ragu pizza quick sauce
½ large tomato sliced
½ red and green pepper sliced
2 handfuls fresh spinach
¼ onion chopped
½ cup mushrooms
½ cup shredded carrots or broccoli slaw
2 oz. Canadian bacon (optional)
1 cup mozzarella cheese

Use Mama Mary's pizza crust (Thin crust). Layer with pizza sauce, onions, fresh spinach, shredded carrots or broccoli slaw, fresh tomatoes, mushrooms, garlic (optional), Canadian bacon mozzarella cheese and bake at 350 for approx. 12 minutes. Cut into 8 slices. 2 slices is the appropriate portion size.

WILTED SPINACH

3-4 cups fresh spinach
½ can Rotel Tomatoes
1oz. feta cheese

Sauté fresh spinach and add ½ can of rotel tomatoes. Season spinach with salt and pepper and sprinkle in 1oz. feta cheese.

AMAZING POWER OF FOOD TOP FOOD LIST
FOR VITAMINS AND MINERALS

VITAMIN A- Responsible for healthy eyes, healthy skin, and good resistance to infection.

1 cup apricots
1 cup beets
1 cup bok choy
1 cup broccoli
½ cantaloupe
1 large carrot
1 cup of kale
1 cup spinach
1 sweet potato
1 cup mixed vegetables

B COMPLEX- Helps the body metabolize protein, carbohydrates, and fats and in the production of cells, blood, and nerve fiber endings. Helps alleviate depression and helps body produce serotonin, an important brain chemical.

1/2 cup soy beans
1 cup spinach
1 cup chick peas
Whole wheat
1 cup lentils
4 oz. salmon
3 oz. hamburger
1 cup kidney beans
1 cup low fat yogurt
1 cup carrots

VITAMIN C – Aids in iron absorption, metabolism of folate and proteins, heals wounds, "holds" cells together, and when a cold appears, it helps you feel better sooner.

1 cup broccoli
1 cup cooked cabbage
1 cup mangos
½ grapefruit
1 orange
1 cup cooked spinach
5 oz. strawberries
1 cup asparagus
1 cup cauliflower
1 cup sweet potato

VITAMIN D – Helps calcium absorption and the onset of osteoporosis. Calcium would not be able to do its job effectively without vitamin D.

4 oz. salmon
1 oz. dry cereals
1 cup milk
4 oz. sardines
4 oz. tuna
4 oz. mackerel
Sunlight

POTASSIUM – Helps to keep muscles and nerves functioning, in synthesizing protein and in storing carbohydrates.

1 cup lima beans
1 cup navy beans
1 potato
4 oz. fresh salmon
½ cup soybeans
5 prunes
1 tomato
1 cup lentils
½ cup pumpkin seeds
4 oz. packed tuna

ZINC – It's a part of certain enzymes and helps in making protein and building bones. Zinc affects the senses of smell and taste and aids in healing wounds. Zinc deficiency symptoms can be poor appetite, suboptimal growth, hair loss, fatigue, and reduced resistance to infections.

1 cup brown rice
4 oz. salmon
]1 cup spinach
1 oz shredded wheat
4 oz. turkey meat
1 tablespoon wheat germ
1 cup low fat yogurt
1 cup crabmeat
4 oz. lean beef
1 cup cottage cheese

CALCIUM – Linked to heart health, cancer prevention and better bones.

1 cup milk
1 cup mustard greens
1 cup broccoli
1 cup beets
1 cup soybeans
1 cup plain yogurt
1 cup okra
½ cup oysters
4 oz. tofu
1 cup bok choy

MAGNESIUM – Essential to the nervous system and its possible magnesium has an important role in preventing heart disease.

1 cup kidney beans
1 cup broccoli
1 cup carrots
4 oz. chicken
1 cup corn
1 baked potato
1 cup blackberries
1 medium banana
1 cup celery
½ cup dates

I have been unbelievably blessed to work with many people over the years, and I could tell you one success story after another. I have seen people lose hundreds of pounds and others run marathons when they had never run a day in their life. I have witnessed the Amazing Power of Food program help people eliminate all daily medications, which has lead them to live excellent, healthy lives. The power of nutrition can help people overcome and avoid disease. In fact, it will help you not only survive, but thrive. It can happen for you, too. Give healthy eating a real chance to change your life. It will. Here are just a few testimonies that may help:

PROOF IS IN THE PUDDING:

"My health was on a decline, I felt very sluggish and had no energy. My physical appearance had changed since I was younger. After my son was born, my health became more important to me and I wanted to do everything I could to be around for him. My doctors had already told me that I was headed for a heart attack or stroke.

"Week one I felt better. My energy was way better. I lost 2lbs the first week and my weight kept dropping the longer I used the menus and theories behind the APF program. It pushed me past my plateau. I went to bed feeling satisfied, but not full. I never felt really hungry. After 6 weeks the doctor wanted me to totally get off of cholesterol medicine completely.

-Chris Bankston
Age 41

PROOF IS IN THE PUDDING:

"I found it very easy to follow and, in fact, it was more food than I was eating during my 'self-dieting' period. It was just a combination of different foods to better fuel my body for the work out regiment I was doing. The most surprising aspect of the program has been that I seldom feel hungry and I feel great!"

-Ronnie Fugarino
Age 52
Lost 10 lbs and 9 inches in 10 weeks

PROOF IS IN THE PUDDING:

"I have lost over 150 pounds in the last year and a half by committing to exercise every day and following the Amazing Power of Food. My energy level is much higher. I feel like I have more endurance and I just feel better. I am no longer taking any cholesterol medicine. My journey has been amazing and I feel amazing."

-Tim Naquin
Age 35
Lost 150lbs. in one year

PROOF IS IN THE PUDDING:

"When I worked with Julie she literally broke out a calculator and added up this little bit here and this glass of wine and that glass of wine...it adds up really quick."

-Geri O'Krepki
Age 46
Lost 20 lbs in 8 weeks

PROOF IS IN THE PUDDING:

"As my weight started to go down, my friends wanted to know more. I described some of my favorite food changes and told them that I now know that every bite of food makes a difference....Julie's advice is common sense, not fad dieting."

-Kathy Blomquist
Age 57

© T h e A m a z i n g P o w e r o f F o o d

Daily Food Log

Date: _____   Su M Tu W Th F Sa

Time	Qty	Food	Calories	Fat

Total: [|]

Water (1 cup per circle)

O O O O O O O O O O O O O O O O

1 cup = 8 fluid oz. = 0.24 liters

Daily Food Log

Date: _____   Su M Tu W Th F Sa

Time	Qty	Food	Calories	Fat

Total: _____ _____

Water (1 cup per circle)

O O O O O O O O O O O O O O O O

1 cup = 8 fluid oz. = 0.24 liters

Daily Food Log

Date: _____

Time	Qty	Food	Calories	Fat

Total:

Water (1 cup per circle)

O O O O O O O O O O O O O O O

1 cup = 8 fluid oz. = 0.24 liters

Daily Food Log

Date: _____   Su M Tu W Th F Sa

Time	Qty	Food	Calories	Fat
		Total:		

Water (1 cup per circle)

O O O O O O O O O O O O O O O O O

1 cup = 8 fluid oz. = 0.24 liters

© The Amazing Power of Food

We hope you enjoyed this book. For additional meal plans and more
information please contact:

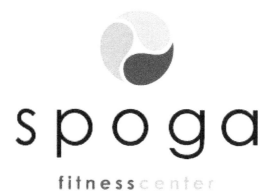

spoga

fitness center

811 CM Fagan Drive
Hammond, Louisiana 70401

Email: amazingpoweroffood@gmail.com
Web: www.powerfoodsco.com
Phone: 985.345.2453

This book is also available at
www.amazon.com
www.spogafc.com

Made in the USA
Columbia, SC
16 June 2018